25% OFF Online Medical-Surgical Nurse Prep Course!

Dear customer,

We consider it an honor and a privilege that you chose our Medical-Surgical Nurse Study Guide. As a way of showing our appreciation and to help us better serve you, we have partnered with Mometrix Test Preparation to offer **25% off their online Med-Surg Prep Course**. Many online prep courses are needlessly expensive and don't deliver enough value. With their course, you get access to the best Medical-Surgical Nurse prep material, and you only pay 3/4 of the price.

Mometrix has structured their online course to perfectly complement your printed study guide. The Med-Surg Prep Course contains **in-depth lessons** that cover all the most important topics, **video reviews** that explain difficult concepts, over **800 practice questions to ensure you feel prepared, and more than** 300 digital flashcards, so you can study while you're on the go.

Online Medical-Surgical Nurse Prep Course

Topics Covered	Course Features
Assessment and Diagnosis • Physical Assessment, Laboratory Testing, and More	**Medical-Surgical Nurse Study Guide** • Get content that complements our best-selling study guide.
Planning, Implementation, and Evaluation • Patient Education, Dialysis, and More	**Full-Length Practice Tests and Flashcards** • With over 800 practice questions and 300+ digital flashcards, You can test yourself again and again
Professional Role • Therapeutic Communication, Nursing Ethics, and More	**Mobile friendly** • If you need to study on the go, the course is easily accessible From your mobile device.

To receive this discount, visit their website at **bit.ly/surgnursecourse** or simply scan this QR code with your smartphone. At the checkout page, enter the discount code: **HP25**

If you have any questions or concerns, please contact them at **universityhelp@ mometrix.com**

SCAN HERE

CMSRN Exam
Prep
2021-2022

A Medical Surgical Nursing Study Guide with Test Bank
Including 600 Practice Questions and Answers
(Med Surg Certification Review Book)

SHIRLEY WILCHER

Contents

Introduction

Thank you for investing in this content! You have chosen to prepare for a test that could have a significant impact on your future, and this guide is intended to assist you in being properly prepared for test day. You must have a thorough comprehension of the exam subject, but you must also be prepared for the test's particular setting and stressors to perform to the best of your abilities.

We urge that you begin studying for your exam as soon as possible. If you've purchased this book as a last-minute study resource and just have a few days until your test, we recommend skipping the first two Secret Keys because they deal with a long-term study strategy.

If you suffer from test anxiety, we strongly advise you to read through our suggestions for overcoming them. Test anxiety is a strong foe, but it can be defeated, and we want to make sure you have the resources you need.

- Make broad plans and start small.
- Gather and organize your data.
- Make good use of your time.
- Make sure you're recalling the concepts by choosing the correct study setting and the proper time of day to study.
- Select a study strategy that is appropriate for your learning type.
- Take it slowly.
- Make a strategy for guessing.
- Understand how to filter down your options.
- Carefully read the question and the answer options.

- Look for hints in the context.
- Avoid falling into factual traps. Don't get sidetracked by an answer option that is technically correct but doesn't respond to the question.
- Don't waste time if a question appears to be too complex. just move on!
- Please double-check your work. Take a moment to review your answer choices and make sure you've chosen the proper one.
- Calm down and keep going at the speed you've set for yourself.
- Take your time. When you're in a rush, it's quite easy to make mistakes.
- Panic will not assist you in passing the exam. So try to maintain your composure and keep progressing.

Chapter One: **Assessment**

The Nursing Process

The nursing evaluation examines patient information to aid in diagnosis and therapy. To ensure the patient's safety, the nurse evaluates the patient's baseline health and medical history. The nurse also determines whether the patient has any difficulties in terms of comprehension or cooperation.

The goal of nursing diagnosis is to improve the patient's comfort and outcome. Nurses use a diagnosis to determine which nursing interventions are required to keep the patient safe and comfortable. The diagnosis is used by the nurse to administer therapy and anticipate possible actions.

The nurse can plan out the methodologies, nursing responsibilities, possible interventions, and expected outcomes needed to meet the patient's objectives.

The nursing plan must be implemented with some flexibility, and the original plan may be updated as the plan progresses to reflect the patient's particular needs. The records might also be used for legal and research purposes.

The nurse must assess procedures and actions in connection to standards of care, quality of care, and patient outcomes to offer the greatest care for the patient.

Compilation of Medical Records

Nursing care needs are identified through a health history assessment and a system evaluation. In a nursing health history, various elements must be included:

- The biographical component
- The main problem
- The current illness's history
- History of medical treatment
- History of the family
- System evaluation
- Patient's way of life
- History of social life
- Psychological condition
- Methods of receiving health-care services.

Physical Examination

When doing a nursing assessment, it is critical to understand the typical structure and function of anatomy and physiology across the patients' lifetime, from neonates to geriatric. Lungs, kidneys, heart, adrenal glands, pituitary, and parathyroid are examples of homeostatic organs.

To maintain fluid and electrolyte balance, the body's fluid additions and losses should be roughly equal daily. Intake and output can be measured to keep track of this (I & O).

Physical evaluations should be planned and systematic, as well as age and developmentally appropriate. A thorough physical exam or a system-specific exam may be performed.

Inspection, palpation, auscultation, and percussion are the four main procedures used in a physical exam.

Assessment of the Cardiovascular System

Questioning the patient about any family history of death at a young age or other cardiovascular disorders is part of the cardiovascular examination. Edema, chest pain, dyspnea, weariness, vertigo, syncope or other changes in consciousness, weight gain, and leg cramps or pain should all be discussed with the patient. Vital signs, heart and lung sounds, skin examination, radial, popliteal, and pedal pulses, circulation and sensation of extremities, and auscultation of the aorta, renal, iliac, and femoral arteries for bruits are all part of the physical examination.

Assessment of the Respiratory System

If the patient is in severe respiratory distress, it is necessary to stabilize the patient before taking a respiratory history or asking family members if they are available. Assess vital signs, posture, pulse oximetry, check nails for clubbing, do a skin evaluation, listen to lung sounds via auscultation and percussion, and look for auxiliary muscle use, symptoms of anxiety, and edema when completing a physical evaluation. Blood may be obtained for arterial blood gases, electrolytes, and CBC tests, depending on the patient's condition. It is possible to get sputum cultures.

Assessment of the Endocrine System

Changes in these areas are suggestive of endocrine diseases since the endocrine system includes organs that manufacture hormones that are crucial to growth, sexual development, and metabolism. While symptoms can vary, most endocrine disorders have a set of symptoms that might be associated with them. Fatigue and capacity to do ADLs, heat or cold intolerance, changes in sexual drive, sexual functioning, and secondary sexual features, weight fluctuation, sleep problems, impaired attention and memory, and mood changes should all be discussed with the patient. During the physical examination, look for edema, a "moon" face or "buffalo hump," exophthalmos, hair loss, feminine facial hair, a comparatively large trunk with thin extremities, and relatively large hands and feet.

Assessment of Neurological System

Examine the patient's medical history for signs of trauma, falls, alcoholism, drug misuse, current medications, and a family history of neurological issues. Inquire about any presenting neurological symptoms, including seizures, pain, vertigo, weakness, abnormal sensations, visual problems, loss of consciousness, changes in cognition, and motor problems, as well as the circumstances in which they occur, whether they fluctuate, and any associated factors, such as seizures, pain, vertigo, weakness, abnormal sensations, visual problems, loss of consciousness, changes in cognition, and motor problems.

Assessment of the Digestive System

Inquire about personal and family history of gastrointestinal issues, as well as risk factors like alcoholism, smoking, drug and prescription usage, and bad eating habits. Inquire about GI discomfort, flatus, nausea, vomiting, diarrhea, and abdominal pain, among other symptoms. Determine the pattern of defecation and inquire about weight swings.

When completing a physical examination, examine the oral mucosa, tongue, teeth, throat, thyroid and parathyroid glands, skin color, moisture, turgor, nodules or lesions, bruises, scars, abdominal shape, and bowel sounds, using the stethoscope diaphragm to assess the abdomen in all four quadrants.

- **Gallbladder and Pancreatic Disease Evaluation.** The emergence of symptoms prompts gallbladder and pancreatic evaluations. Gallbladder disease causes epigastric discomfort after eating fatty foods, as well as abdominal distention. Pain in the right upper quadrant, which may be colicky, nausea, and vomiting are all possible symptoms. Intermittent pain is possible. Pancreatitis can cause significant abdominal discomfort, back pain, significant vomiting, and dyspnea in the patient. Pancreatitis is frequently linked to gallstones or alcoholism, so a history of alcohol consumption and a gallstone examination is required.
- **Evaluation for Liver Disease.** Before lab tests reveal abnormalities, the liver must be 70% destroyed. To detect early disease, risk factors and early symptoms must be assessed. Alcoholism and drug misuse,

hazardous sexual activities, infection or exposure to environmental contaminants, and travel to countries with poor sanitation are all risk factors for liver disease. Questions about exhaustion, itching, abdominal pain, anorexia, weight gain, fever, blood in the stools or black feces, sleep issues, lack of menstruation, and libido should be asked of the patient. Examining vital signs and the skin for scratches, pallor, jaundice, dryness, bruises, petechiae, abdominal veins and spider angiomas, and red palms are all part of the physical examination.

Assessment of the Genitourinary System

Examine the patient's medical history for family history of urinary system disease and risk factors such as past urinary system disease, advanced age, and immobility. Hypertension, diabetes, chemical exposure, chronic disease, pelvic radiation, STDs, alcohol or drug use, and pregnancy and delivery problems are all factors to consider.

Determine daily fluid intake and inquire about symptoms like flank or abdominal pain, hesitancy, urgency, difficulty or straining with voiding, difficulty emptying the bladder, urinary incontinence, fatigue, SOB, anemia-related exercise intolerance, fever, chills, blood in the urine, and GI symptoms.

Vital signs, kidney and bladder palpation, and percussion over the bladder after urination are all part of the physical examination.

Musculoskeletal Assessment

An evaluation to determine the mechanism of harm in a musculoskeletal injury.

- **Question/Audience Participation:** The patient (if alert and cognizant), family or friends, and first responders may typically determine how, when, and where an injury occurred. In some circumstances, police reports may be available. Any information presented should be clarified by the trauma nurse by asking questions.
- **Observation:** The patient's overall appearance (clean, soiled, unkempt,

well-dressed, sporting clothes/uniform), visible injuries (bruises, swelling, and bleeding), and odor (fruity, alcohol, urine, feces) may reveal information about the mechanism of injury or the patient's general health and living situation.

- **Physical Examination:** The trauma nurse should look for common damage patterns linked with various injury mechanisms. A fall from a great height, for example, can result in both foot and back fractures. Falls frequently result in hip and wrist fractures. Blistering, redness, and tissue sloughing are all signs of burns.

Integumentary Evaluation

Ethnicity has an impact on skin tone. Color changes should be evaluated to see if they are localized or widespread, as well as if they are permanent or transitory. Stress, poor oxygenation, and vasoconstriction can all cause a pale complexion. Vasodilation, local inflammation, and flushing are all signs of erythema. Jaundice suggests elevated bilirubin and cyanosis implies poor oxygenation.

Temperature is usually measured by touching the back of the hand to the skin. The skin should be warm and even on both sides. Hypothermia can be caused by poor circulation, intravenous infusion, or a paralyzed limb (such as in a cast). Fever, infection, and excessive exercise can cause hyperthermia.

Pain assessment

- **Nociceptors.** The main neurons, or sensory receptors, in the skin, muscle, and joints, as well as the stomach, bladder, and uterus, respond to stimuli. Mechanical, thermal, and chemical stimuli elicit specialized responses in these neurons.
- **Nociceptive Pain.** Pain induced by neuroreceptor activation is referred to as nociceptive pain. This stimulation occurs as a result of tissue damage. Internal organs are related to visceral pain. Messages from pain receptors in the cutaneous or musculoskeletal tissues are referred to as somatic pain.
- **Neuropathic pain.** Neuropathic pain is caused by a neural system in-

jury. This can be caused by cancer cells crushing the nerves or spinal cord, by true malignant invasion into the nerves or spinal cord, or by chemotherapy and radiation causing chemical damage to the nerves.

Geriatric Evaluation

The elderly can be categorized into three categories. The young-old are defined as those between the ages of 65 and 74. The middle-aged are those aged 75 to 84, and the old-old are those aged 85 and up. As a person progresses through these age categories, significant physical and psychological changes occur. As the population grows, so does the number of people suffering from physical and mental disorders.

Psychosocial Evaluation

A psychological assessment, in addition to the physical exam, should provide extra information to assist the patient's treatment approach, including the following:

- Previous hospitalizations and healthcare experience
- **Psychiatric background:** Suicidal ideation, psychiatric illnesses, a family history of psychiatric illness, a history of violence, and/or self-mutilation are all factors to consider.
- **The main complaint:** The patient's perspective
- **Complementary and alternative therapies:** Acupuncture, visualization, and meditation are three techniques that can help you relax.
- **Background in both work and education:** Work, retirement, and specialized talents
- Family and friends, living circumstances, regular hobbies, and support systems are all examples of social patterns.
- **Sexual inclinations:** Orientation, issues, and sex customs
- **Interests and skills:** Sports and hobbies
- **Substance misuse, current or previous:** Type, frequency, a pattern of drinking, recreational drug usage, and prescription drug overuse
- **Ability to cope:** Techniques for reducing stress
- **Physical, sexual, emotional, and financial abuse:** Seniors are particu-

larly vulnerable to these forms of abuse and may be hesitant to report them out of shame or fear.

- **Spiritual/cultural evaluation:** Religious/spiritual significance, practices, and prohibitions (such as blood products or foods) as well as their impact on health and health decisions

Assessment of Cognitive Ability

People with dementia, delirium, or short-term memory loss should have their cognition tested. Both the mini-mental state examination (MMSE) and the mini-cog test are widely employed. These tests entail the individual performing specific tasks and serve as a baseline for determining changes in mental health.

Neglect and Abuse

Any symptoms that may indicate a possibility for or an actual situation involving abuse should always be kept in mind by the nurse. These indicators could be found in the patient's medical history. The following are some examples of indicators concerning their primary complaint: a vague description of the problem's cause, inconsistencies between physical findings and explanations, minimizing injuries, a long period between injury and treatment, and family members' over- or under-reactions to injuries. Other crucial information, including a family history of violence, time spent in jail or prison, and a family history of violent deaths or substance misuse, may be revealed in the family genome. Previous injuries, spontaneous abortions, or a history of inpatient mental treatment or substance misuse may all be part of the patient's medical history.

Actual or potential abuse signs can be discovered during the collecting of the patient's medical history, financial history, family values, and connections with family members.

Chapter Two: **Diagnostics**

Diagnostics of the Cardiovascular System

- CK and CK-MB, as well as Troponin I and T, are cardiac enzymes.
- basic "2D Echo," the transesophageal (TEE) probe, doppler imaging, and bubble study are all types of echocardiography.
- EKG testing (EET) and exercise imaging testing (exercise, or "stress" echocardiography, and exercise myocardial perfusion imaging) are two types of stress echocardiography.

Diagnostics of the Endocrine System

- Glucose test in the lab
- HHaemoglobinA1C test in the lab
- Thyroid function testing and antibody testing are both basic tests.

Diagnostics in Hematology

- WBC Count AND DIFFERENTIAL
- C-REACTIVE PROTEIN AND ERYTHROCYTE SEDIMEN-TATION RATE
- BLood CELLS: hemoglobin, hematocrit, mean corpuscular volume (MCV), and reticulocyte count

Diagnostics in Neurology

- Puncture of the lumbar spine
- The test of Queckenstedt

Gastrointestinal Diagnostics

- Liver function studies: bilirubin, total protein, prothrombin time (PT), alkaline phosphatase, AST (SGOT), ALT (SGPT),
- GGT (GGTP), LDH, Serum ammonia Cholesterol.
- Nutritional laboratory monitoring: total protein, albumin, prealbumin, transferrin, esophagogastroduodenoscopy (EGD)

Diagnostics of the Genitourinary System

- Studies on renal function: osmolality (urine), osmolality (serum), uric acid, creatinine clearance (24-hour), serum creatinine, urine creatinine, blood urea nitrogen (BUN), BUN/creatinine ratio urinalysis is a type of urine analysis.
- Urinalysis: Color, odor specific gravity, pH, sediment, glucose, ketones, protein, blood, bilirubin, nitrate, and Urobilinogen
- Renal scan with IVP and radionucleotide
- Biopsy of the renal system
- Ultrasound for the renal system

Chapter Three: **Planning, Implementation, and Evaluation**

Nursing Care Planning for Patients

With the support of the patient and family, the nursing diagnoses are used to prioritize the patient's needs:

- The patient's priorities and Maslow's Hierarchy of Needs are used to prioritize the needs.
- Each diagnosis has a set of desired outcomes.
- Patient and family involvement is used to develop goals for each nursing diagnosis.
- Each goal is then followed by a list of precise actions that must be taken to attain it.

Prevention and Management of Postoperative Complications

Assisting patients with post-surgery body image issues

Patients who are anticipating change should be allowed to speak with their doctors about the changes and what they mean to them. To reduce feelings of helplessness, patients should have as much choice in their care as possible:

- Assist patients in continuing their normal activities and discussing their feelings with their family and friends.
- Allow patients to express their emotions by providing opportunities for them to do so.
- Encourage patients to do as much as possible for themselves and to accept help when needed
- Provide resources for cosmetics, wigs, special clothing, or prosthesis as needed
- Educate and provide information
- Provide referrals to a counselor or group dealing with the same problems, as this may be helpful
- Provide immediate interventions to complications

Thromboembolism Prevention

Smoking abstinence, regular exercise, birth control pill discontinuation, early ambulation following surgery, SCDs/compression hose, high blood pressure control, peripheral vascular disease treatment, and avoiding extended sitting are all recommended.

Common Viral Pathogens and Their Prevention in Transplant Patients

- Primary transmission can be prevented through serologic matching, however, due to the scarcity of organs, this may be difficult.

- Early detection using serum testing allows for more targeted treatment.
- Antiviral prophylaxis can be useful in high-risk patients.
- Immunization has been shown to be both safe and effective in reducing the incidence and severity of infection.
- Immunoglobulin is provided to transplant recipients who have been exposed to specific viruses.
- If feasible, reduce immunosuppressive medicines.
- For some viruses, high-dose acyclovir may help to lessen the severity of infection.
- The most practicable strategies of infection control are to target people at the highest risk of disease through surveillance and to use effective transmission-based measures.

After Transplant Surgery, Preventing Common Bacterial Infections

- In these patients, handwashing and basic cleaning techniques remain the most effective ways of infection management.
- Antibiotic prophylaxis and environmental monitoring are both beneficial.

Prevention of Aspergillus Fungal Infection after Transplant Surgery

- High-risk patients are to have rooms with laminar airflow or HEPA filtration to improve air filtration and their environment must also be monitored.
- Guidelines must be followed to ensure that debris and dust from construction do not get to the patient's wards.
- To begin treatment with the drug of choice (voriconazole), standard precautions of diagnosing early with high-resolution CT scans instead of chest x-rays should be followed.

Prevention of Infection Control Strategies for Spinal Cord Injuries

- **Urinary tract infection:** Patients should be checked regularly symptoms of infection such as changes in spasm, fever, or voiding habits. Sterile intermittent catheterization should be used when in the hospital, instead of continuous catheterization.
- **Antibiotic prophylaxis** hasn't produced positive results except for bacterial interference, positive responses has been seen when colonizing the urinary tract by making use of nonpathogenic £. coli 83972.
- **Decubital ulcers:** It is important to turn patients, monitor the condition of the skin, and prevent the development of pressure by avoiding friction. The patients and staff must be taught about cleanliness, prevention, and skincare. The skin's integrity must be maintained with enough hydration and nutrition.
- **Respiratory infections:** The ventilation equipment must be properly used. infections can be reduced by assisted coughing that is through postural drainage and respiratory therapy. Patients are to get pneumonia immunization although the use of prophylactic antibiotics is not recommended.

Chapter Four: **Cardiovascular**

Cardiovascular Pathophysiology

Acute Coronary Syndromes

This arises as a result of the coronary arteries having inadequate blood flow which causes ischemia of the cardiac muscle. Angina occurs regularly in acute coronary syndrome causing a crushing pain around the sternum moving down the left arm or even both arms. Although symptoms may not be as severe in the elderly, diabetics, and females and may include fatigue, nausea, shortness of breath, weakness/numbness/ pain in the arms, or no pain that is the ischemia is silent.

Myocardial Infarctions

- **Non-ST-segment elevation MI (NSTEMI):** On the electrocardiogram ECG), the ST elevates due to myocardial damage occurring from severe ischemia or infarction.
- **ST-segment elevation MI (STEMI):** This MI is more severe as it causes total blockage of one or more coronary arteries coupled with myocardial damage which causes the ST to be elevated.

- **Q-Wave AND Non-Q-Wave Myocardial Infarctions.**

○ Q-Wave is evident by the various abnormal Q waves which are wider and deeper on the ECG, particularly early in the morning which can be linked to adrenergic activity. Infarction mostly occurs for a long time and leads to necrosis. It is mostly but not transmural all the time.

○ Non-Q-Wave is evident when the ST- T wave changes with ST depression and it can usually be reversed in a few days. Reperfusion can occur randomly which causes its infarct size to be smaller. It's mostly non-transmural.

Myocardial infarctions can be categorized by the severity of the injury and its location. The way myocardial infarctions occur clinically differs significantly. The following ECG which monitors the changes in the heart are Labs (Creatinine kinase (CK-MB), Myoglobin, Troponin, and Ischemia Modified Albumin (IMA)) and Echocardiogram and are used for proper diagnosis.

Aortic Aneurysms

When the aorta's wall is torn and the layers between the wall dilate and weaken till it risks a split, it's called a dissecting aortic aneurysm which has a mortality rate of 90%. While AAA is usually due to atherosclerosis it could also arise due to connective tissue disorders, Marfan syndrome, and Ehlers-Danlos disease. It could also be classified as Types I, II, & III according to DeBakey classification which uses anatomic location. TEE/transthoracic echocardiogram, X-ray, cardiac catheterization, MRI, and CT can be used to diagnose. The use of Intubation and ventilation, Surgical repair (Open or Endovascular), Anti-hypertensives and Analgesia/sedation can be used to treat it.

- **Aortic Rupture.** Aortic rupture occurs due to rupture or trauma to the aortic aneurysm and it leads to the dangerous breakage of the aorta. The aortic rupture that occurs randomly is mostly in the abdominal aorta.
- **Cardiogenic Shock.** Cardiogenic shock occurs when the body does not get enough oxygen or blood for adequate circulation when the heart does not pump blood adequately.
- **Obstructive shock.** Obstructive shock is a result of the preload, that

is, the diastolic filling of the RV is blocked in one or more ways. Important vessels of the heart like the pulmonary embolism could be obstructed which causes excessive afterload and this leads to a decrease in cardiac output or there could be a reduction of the heart as a result of air or blood filling the pericardial sac with tension pneumothorax or cardiac tamponade.

- **Cardiac Tamponade.** Pericardial effusion occurs with Cardiac tamponade and it applies pressure on the heart. It could arise due to pericarditis, heart failure, trauma, pneumothorax, or cardiac surgery. To limit friction, the pericardial area must have about 50ML of fluid circulating it and if there is a sudden rise in the air or volume present in the pericardial sac, it could lead to various cardiac responses due to the heart being compressed.

Cardiomyopathy

Dilated Cardiomyopathy. This results in decreased cardiac perfusion due to some precipitating factors. It causes the scar tissue to replace the arising ischemic cardiac tissue and this forces the healthy cells to be overworked leading to overstretching and hypertrophy. This then ultimately makes the muscle cells unable to contract as they have been overstretched leading to weak chamber and dilation. It reduces the cardiac output and stroke volume causing severe valve regurgitation, enlargement of the mitral, as well as tricuspid valves

Hypertrophic Cardiomyopathy. This is a result of a genetic disorder, which involves mainly parts of the left ventricle and the ventricular septum, causing the heart muscle to thicken. Those with HCM are characterized by misalignment of muscle cells or myocardial disarray and produce abnormal sarcomeres. HCM comes with a variety of symptoms like myocardial disarray, ventricular hypertrophy, cardiac dysrhythmias, an asymmetrical septum, and forceful systole. Due to the abnormal cells taking a long time to develop, HCM is commonly not diagnosed until middle or late adulthood.

Restrictive Cardiomyopathy. This arises as a result of ventricular becoming non-compliant which causes a reduction in the volume of end-diastolic cardiac refill. The stiffening of the ventricles is a result of the cardiac muscle being infiltrated with the fibroelastic tissue as seen in the case of sarcoidosis or amyloidosis.

Dysrhythmias

- **Sinus Bradycardia.** SB occurs when the rate of impulse from the sinus node is decreased. Apart from showing at a slower rate, the ECG and the pulse would usually appear normal.
- **Sinus Tachycardia. ST** is a result of an increase in the frequency of the sinus node impulse. It usually shows a steady pulse of >100 with P waves before QRS although it could also be part of the preceding T wave.
- **Supraventricular Tachycardia.** Supraventricular tachycardia (SVT) (>100 BPM) could lead to congestive heart failure due to sudden onset. Cardiac output could reduce greatly as filling time decreases due to the rate increasing to 200-300 BMP.
- **Sinus Arrhythmia.** SA occurs when the sinus node gets irregular impulses, usually paradoxical which increase with inspiration and decrease with expiration. It occurs during inspiration while stimulating the vagal nerve and it hardly results in a hemodynamic effect being negative.

Atrial Dysrhythmias

- **Premature Atrial Contractions.** This is an extra beat before the sinus impulse which is caused by an electrical impulse aimed at the atrium.
- **Atrial Flutter.** This is when the atrial rate beats at 250-400 beats per minute which is faster than the rate the AV node conducts so not every beat is conducted into the ventricles.
- **Atrial Fibrillation.** This is as a result of unorganized and hurried beats that cannot empty the atria which causes blood to pool into the chamber. This causes emboli and thrombus.

Premature Junctional Contractions. PJCs are as a result of a premature impulse starting at the AV node prior to the next normal sinus getting to the AV node. They are identical to premature atrial contractions and usually don't need treatment even though they do not indicate digoxin toxicity.

Junctional Rhythms. This is when the heart uses the AV node as its pacemaker. This occurs due to the sinus node depressing from an increased vagal tone or the AV node being blocked which doesn't allow the sinus impulse to be transmitted.

AV Nodal Reentry Tachycardia. This is the result of an impulse being conducted to the AV node's section and is then directed back in a fast repeated cycle to the same section as well as the ventricular which causes a rapid ventricular rate. The beginning and end are usually fast.

Premature Ventricular Contractions. They are in which the impulse begins and conducts through the ventricles before the sinus impulse is about to come. Ectopic QRS complexes could come different in shape, and it's determined if there is one (unifocal site) or more (multifocal site) that induces ectopic beats.

Ventricular Tachycardia. This is having 3 PVCs and giving 100-200 beats per minute of ventricular rate. It may be caused by the same circumstances as PVC and is usually associated with underlying coronary artery disease. It is very dangerous as the rate of contraction is too fast as those ineffective beats may make the patient lose consciousness without having a noticeable pulse.

Ventricular Fibrillation. This is characterized by an irregular and fast ventricular rate of >300 beats per minute without any atrial activity showing on the ECG, this arises due to the ventricles having disorganized electrical activity. Due to the ECG showing irregular undulations, the QRS complex is not noticeable.

Idioventricular Rhythm. This is as a result of the Purkinje fibers creating an impulse beneath the AV node. It could be due to a blockage at the AV node or if the sinus node doesn't fire which prevents the impulse from passing through.

Ventricular Asystole. This is also called cardiac arrest and it is the absence of palpable pulse, audible heartbeat, and respiration. At first, the ECG may present some P waves, there would be no QRS complex even if there may be few QRS escape beats or agonal rhythms.

Sinus Pause. This arises when the sinus node doesn't function appropriately while stimulating the contraction heart which causes there to be a pause in the ECG recording which may last for some seconds to minutes and it depends on how severe the dysfunction is. It may be difficult to identify a long pause from a cardiac arrest.

First-Degree AV Block. This arises when the atrial impulses are carried out at a rate slower than normal through the AV node to the ventricles.

Second-Decree AV Block. Blockage of some of the atrial beats is known as second-degree AV block. It can be divided into block patterns Mobitz type I and II.

Third-Degree AV Block. This allows more P waves than QRS complexes without a definite relationship between them. The PR interval is irregular as the atrial rate exceeds the pulse rate by 2-3 times.

Bundle Branch Blocks. This is as a result of conduction in the right bundle branch being blocked as it carries impulses to the right ventricle from the bundle. The impulse then goes to the left ventricle before getting to the right ventricle, although this delays contraction of the right ventricle.

Heart Failure. Heart failure (formerly congestive heart failure) is a cardiac disease that includes disorders of contractions (systolic dysfunction) or filling (diastolic dysfunction) or both and may melude pulmonary, peripheral, or systemic edema. The most common causes are coronary artery disease, systemic or pulmonary hypertension. cardiomyopathy, and valvular disorders.

Systolic Heart Failure. This is usually known as the left-sided failure which decreases the amount of blood removed from the ventricles when it contracts (reduced election fraction). This causes the SNS to make catecholamines to helps the myocardium and would lead to down regulation, destruction of adrenergic and beta receptor sites, and eventually more myocardial damage.

Diastolic Heart Failure. It may be hard to distinguish this from systolic heart failure as their symptoms are similar. Diastolic heart failure prevents the myocardium from relaxing properly which would aid in filling the ventricles. This may be what leads to systolic heart failure as myocardial hypertrophy causes the muscles to get stiff and their causes are the same.

Acute Heart Failure. This is a result of the body being unable to make up for the heart's inability to give enough perfusion. The metabolic demands of the body are then not met as cardiac output is not enough anymore. Acute heart failure arises without warning and can be brought on by illness, fluid overflow, noncompliance with medications, dysrhythmias, acute ischemia, hypertensive crisis, or non-compliance with medications.

Acute Cardiac-Related Pulmonary Edema. It arises when there is heart failure which causes fluid overflow and leads to third-spacing of the fluid to the lung's interstitial spaces. Pulmonary edema could be from mitral stenosis, MI, volume overload, chronic HF, or ischemia.

Hypertensive Crises. They are marked elevations in blood pressure which if not treated, could lead to serious damage to the organs. It may be caused by non-compliance to medication, dissection of aortic aneurysm, stroke, pulmonary edema, pheochromocytoma (endocrine or renal disorder), subarachnoid hemorrhage, and eclampsia. It could be divided into hypertensive urgency and hypertensive emergency.

Endocarditis. This causes the lining of the heart which covers the heat valves to be infected and to contain Purkinje fibers called endocardium. Those at risk are males, those with dental infections, being 60 years of age, and IV drug users . Infective endocarditis's most common source is staphylococcal aureus.

Myocarditis. This is caused by a viral infection like HIV, influenza virus, and Coxsackie virus and it's the inflammation of muscle tissue (cardiac myocardium). Myocarditis could also be a result of an allergic reaction to medications, bacteria, parasites, or fungi. At times, it could arise due to complications of endocarditis. Some antibiotics and chemotherapy drugs could also cause it.

Acute Pericarditis. This is when the pericardial sac is inflamed and it could be with or without an increased pericardial fluid. It could be due to an underlying disease or it may be an isolated process. If the underlying cause is due to any kind of malignancy or autoimmune, the patient tends to exhibit the symptoms related to that disorder.

Mitral Stenosis. This occurs when the mitral valve narrows allowing blood to flow from the left atrium to the left ventricle. To overcome resistance, pressure in the left atrium increases, and this leads to the left atrium being enlarged while also increasing the pressure in pulmonary hypertension (capillaries of the lung) and pulmonary veins. Mitral stenosis arises due to tumors, endocarditis, or calcification in the left atrium.

Mitral Valve Insufficiency. This is as a result of the mitral valve not closing properly causing a backflow to the left atrium from the left ventricle during systole, causing the cardiac output to decrease. It could occur alone or with mitral stenosis. Mitral valve insufficiency could arise due to left heart failure/cardiomyopathy, damage caused by rheumatic fever, infective endocarditis, myxomatous degeneration, or Marfan's syndrome (collagen vascular disease). The three phases of the disease are Acute, Chronic compensated, and Chronic decompensated.

Aortic Stenosis. This occurs when the aortic valve which controls the blood flow from the left ventricle narrows. This increases pressure to overcome the valvular resistance, as the left ventricle thickens, causing the need for the coronary arteries' bloody supply and after load to increase.

Pulmonic Stenosis. This comes up when the pulmonary blood allows the flow of blood from the right ventricle to the lungs to narrow. This may arise without symptoms which make it difficult to diagnose until adulthood depending on how severe it is.

Acute Peripheral Vascular Insufficiency. This is when there is a blockage of a blood vessel which leads to tissue ischemia and finally leads to necrosis and cellular death.

Acute Venous Thromboembolism. This is characterized by pulmonary emboli (PE) and deep vein thrombosis (DVT). Acute venous thromboembolism (VTE) could be a result of inflammation, invasive procedures, and lack of mobility which makes it common in intensive care units.

Cardiovascular Procedures and Interventions

Cardioversion. This is used to send timely electrical stimulation to the heart which turns a tachydysrhythmia like atrial fibrillation back to a normal sinus rhythm.

Emergency Defibrillation. This is used to treat decompensating hemodynamics, pulseless ventricular tachycardia, polymorphic ventricular tachycardia with a rapid rate, and acute ventricular fibrillation by sending in uncoordinated shock.

Pericardiocentesis. This can be done with ultrasound guidance and ECG to ease cardiac tamponade or ultrasound guidance to identify pericardial effusion. Pericardiocentesis could be used to treat cardiac arrest or also preventing PEA from having the pressure of the jugular venous increased.

Pacemakers. They are used to help the heart perform its expected conduction system when the heart is faulty. Pacemaker could be used temporarily or inserted permanently.

- Temporary transvenous pacemakers
- Epicardial pacing.
- Transcutaneous pacing.

Automatic ICD. This is like a pacemaker and it is also inserted similarly by one or more leads going to the epicardium or the ventricular myocardium, although it is used to control fibrillation and/or tachycardia.

Central Line Insertion. This allows CVP measuring, blood testing, and fast administration of large volumes of fluid.

Intraosseous Infusion. This can be used in place of adult emergencies, pediatric emergencies, and IV access for neonates, when fast and temporary access is needed or when vascular access or peripheral access cannot be accomplished. It is usually used for pediatric cardiac arrest.

Vascular Interventions. This is used for patients with diseases that reduce blood flow to the limbs leading to ischemia-related damage. Diseases requiring vascular interventions include congenital defect, severe unresponsive vascular disease, damaged vessels, acute occlusion/embolus, or ruptured /dissecting aneurysm.

- Aortic Aneurysm Repair
- Embolectomy
- Bypass grafts

Fem-Pop Bypass. This is used to bypass an obstructed femoral artery below or above the knee for femoral artery disease. A vein graft like the saphenous vein or man-made vein is used and sewn below to the popliteal artery or above the occluded area to the femoral artery which allows blood to pass through the blocked area.

Peripheral Stents. This may be used when treating peripheral vascular insufficiency. Peripheral vascular stenting is usually done in interventional radiology where the interventionalist uses balloon angioplasty to remove the vessel beneath fluoroscopic guidance.

Cardiovascular Pharmacology

Anti-Hypertensive Medications. Diuretics, sympatholytics, vasodilators, calcium channel blockers, and angiotensin-converting enzyme inhibitors are the classes of Anti-hypertensive medications used to treat hypertension (ACE inhibitors).

Diuretics. Diuretics improve renal perfusion and filtration, lowering preload and reducing peripheral and pulmonary edema, hypertension, CHF, diabetes insipidus, and obstructive pulmonary disease. Diuretics come in a variety of forms, including loop, thiazide, and potassium-sparing.

Antidysrhythmic Medications. Antidysrhythmic medications are a class of medications that control dysrhythmias by acting on the conduction system, ventricles, and/or atria. Class I, II, III, and IV medications are employed, as well as other unclassified miscellaneous pharmaceuticals having established usefulness in regulating arrhythmias, such as adenosine and electrolyte supplements.

Smooth Muscle Relaxants. Smooth muscle relaxants lower peripheral vascular resistance, however, they can also lead to hypotension and headaches. Sodium nitroprusside (Nipride®), Nitroglycerin (Tridil®), and Hydralazine (Apresoline®) are just a few examples.

Calcium Channel Blockers are drugs that block calcium channels in the body. Calcium channel blockers are arterial vasodilators that can affect both the peripheral and coronary arteries.

Other Vasodilators.

- B-type natriuretic peptide (BNP) (Nesiritide [Natrecor®]) is a non-inotropic vasodilator that is a recombinant form of a human brain peptide. It lowers filling pressure, raises U/0,
- Vasodilation is caused by alpha-adrenergic blockers, which inhibit alpha receptors in arteries and veins.
- Peripheral dilators that impact the renal and mesenteric arteries are selective specific dopamine DA-1-receptor agonists.

Inotropic Agents. Drugs known as inotropic medications are used to boost cardiac output and improve contractility. IV inotropic medicines may raise the risk of death, although they can be utilized if other medications fail. These medications are less effective when taken orally than when given intravenously. B-Adrenergic agonists (Dobutamine and Dopamine) and Phosphodiesterase III inhibitors (Milrinone, Primacor®, and Digoxin, Lanoxin®) are examples of inotropic drugs.

Medications for Heart Failure

- **ACE inhibitors** such as Captopril (Capoten®), enalapril (Vasotec®), and lisinopril (Prinivil®) are used to treat heart failure. Reduce afterload/preload and reverse ventricular remodeling to prevent neuropathy in diabetic patients.
- **Losartan** (Cozaar®) **and valsartan** (Diovan®) are angiotensin receptor blockers (ARBs). Reduce afterload/preload and ventricular remod-

eling, resulting in vasodilation and blood pressure reduction. They're prescribed for people who can't take ACE inhibitors.

- **§-Blockers.** Metoprolol (Lopressor®), carvedilol (Coreg), and esmolol (Brevibloc®) are all examples of beta-blockers. Slowing the heart rate, lowering blood pressure, preventing dysrhythmias, and reversing ventricular remodeling are all things that can be done. Bradyarrhythmia decompensated HF, uncontrolled hypoglycemia/diabetes mellitus, and airway illness are also contraindications.
- **Aldosterone agonist.** Spironolactone (Aldactone®) is an aldosterone agonist. Reduces edema and sodium retention while lowering preload and cardiac hypertrophy, but may raise serum potassium.
- **Furosemide** (Lasix®) is a diuretic that is used to treat congestive heart failure and renal insufficiency. It is used to minimize preload and the inflammatory reaction generated by cardiopulmonary bypass following surgery (post-perfusion syndrome).

Digoxin (LANOXIN®). Digitalis medication is a kind of digoxin, derived from the foxglove plant and is used to improve myocardial contractility, left ventricular output, and slow conduction through the AV node, lowering fast heart rates and facilitating diuresis. Digoxin does not improve mortality; however, it does increase exercise tolerance and lowers heart failure hospitalizations.

Glycoprotein IIB/INA Inhibitors. Glycoprotein IIB/IIA Inhibitors are medications that prevent clots by inhibiting platelet binding before and after invasive cardiac procedures like angioplasty and stent installation. Acute coronary syndromes (ACS) and percutaneous coronary intervention (PCI) are treated with these medications in combination with anticoagulant agents like heparin and aspirin (PCI). Abciximab (ReoPro®), Eptifibatide (Integrilin®), and Tirofiban (Aggrastat®) are all contraindicated in people with a low platelet count or active bleeding.

Pharmacologic Interventions to Improve Perfusion

The goal of pharmacologic measures to improve perfusion is to lower the risk of thromboses:

- Antiplatelet medicines, such as aspirin, Ticlid®, and Plavix®, inhibit clotting by interfering with the function of the plasma membrane. These drugs do not treat clots, but they do prevent blood clots from forming.
- Vasodilators may direct blood away from ischemic areas, however, some such as Pletal®, which dilates arteries and reduces clotting and is used to treat intermittent claudication, may be necessary.
- Antilipemics, such as Zocor® and Questran®, decrease atherosclerosis progression.
- Hemorheology drugs, such as Trental®, reduce fibrinogen, lowering blood viscosity and erythrocyte stiffness; nonetheless, clinical investigations have shown that they are of modest value. It can be used to treat claudication that occurs on a regular basis.
- To improve quality of life, analgesics may be required. In some circumstances, opioids may be required.
- To disintegrate clots, thrombolytics can be injected into a blocked artery under angiography.
- Coumadin® and Lovenox® are anticoagulants that prevent blood clots from forming.

Chapter Five: **Respiratory**

Respiratory Pathophysiology

Acute Pulmonary Embolism (APE)

Acute Pulmonary Embolism is the most serious clinical presentation of venous thrombo-embolism (VTE). It occurs when a pulmonary artery or arteriole is stopped, preventing blood flow to the lungs and thereby causing the oxygenation of the blood. The size of the embolus and the region of blockage determine the clinical symptoms of acute pulmonary embolism (PE).

Preventive interventions for people at risk, including leg exercises, elastic compression stockings, and anticoagulant treatment are the first steps in the medical care of pulmonary embolism.

Acute Lung Injury and Acute Respiratory Distress Syndrome

Acute lung injury (ALI) is a respiratory distress syndrome that leads to acute respiratory distress syndrome (ARDS). ARDS is a potentially lethal respiratory disorder that is always triggered by a lung infection or damage. Acute respiratory distress syndrome (ARDS) is treated by ensuring adequate gas exchange and avoiding further lung damage caused by forced ventilation.

Acute Respiratory Failure (ARF) is a condition in which the lung is unable to either adequately absorb oxygen (i.e., hypoxemia) or excrete carbon dioxide (i.e., hypercarbia).

Tachypnea, tachycardia, anxiety and restlessness, and diaphoresis are the hallmarks/signs of respiratory failure. Symptoms differ depending on the cause. A blockage may generate more noticeable respiratory symptoms than other conditions.

Respiratory Failure in Hypoxemic and Hypercapnic Patients

When the gaseous exchange of oxygen for carbon dioxide cannot keep up with the demand for oxygen or the production of carbon dioxide, hypoxemic respiratory failure develops. Low inhaled oxygen, such as at high elevations or with smoke inhalation, can cause hypoxemic respiratory failure.

Before severe hypoxemia causes irreversible damage to key organs, respiratory failure must be treated urgently.

Pneumonia

Pneumonia is an infection of the lungs. It involves the inflammation of lung parenchyma which causes exudate to fill the alveoli. It is prevalent in both childhood and adulthood. Pneumonia can be a standalone illness or a complication of another infection or condition, such as lung cancer. Bacteria, viruses, parasites, and fungi can all cause pneumonia.

- **Hospital-acquired pneumonia (HAP)** is a kind of Pneumonia caused by hospitalization. It can be defined as pneumonia that appears not to be present at the time of admission but develops at least 48 hours later.
- **Healthcare-associated pneumonia (HCAP)** is pneumonia that develops in a patient within 90 days of being admitted to an acute care hospital or LTAC for two or more days.
- **Ventilator-associated pneumonia (VAP)** is a kind of hospital-ac-

quired pneumonia that occurs more than 48 hours after an ETT is implanted.

- **Pneumonitis/Pneumonia caused by aspiration.** Aspiration pneumonitis/pneumonia can develop from any sort of aspiration. Foreign objects are included. Aspirated material causes an inflammatory response, putting the irritated mucous membrane at increased risk of bacterial infection, which can lead to pneumonia.

Aspiration of a foreign body.

Aspiration of a foreign body can clog the pharynx, larynx, or trachea, resulting in acute dyspnea or asphyxiation, and the object can be dragged distally into the bronchial tree.

Bronchitis (chronic)

Chronic bronchitis is a pulmonary airway illness marked by a severe cough with sputum production for at least three months each year for at least two years. When the airways are irritated (typically by smoke or pollutants), an inflammatory reaction occurs, increasing the number of mucus-secreting glands and goblet cells while ciliary activity declines, resulting in mucus plugging the airways.

Emphysema

Emphysema is a lung disease that affects people of all ages. It is characterized by abnormal distention of air spaces at the ends of terminal bronchioles, as well as degradation of alveolar walls, resulting in less and less gaseous exchange and growing dead space, with hypoxemia, hypercapnia, and respiratory acidosis as a result.

Because COPD cannot be reversed, treatment focuses on delaying its progression, alleviating symptoms, and increasing quality of life:

Chronic ventilatory failure

Chronic ventilatory failure occurs when alveolar ventilation does not increase in response to increased carbon dioxide levels. It is most commonly associated with chronic pulmonary diseases like asthma and COPD, drug overdoses, or diseases that impair respiratory efforts like Guillain-Barré syndrome and myasthenia gravis.

Chronic Asthma

Cough, wheeze, and dyspnea are the three main symptoms of persistent asthma. A strong cough may be the only sign of cough-variant asthma, at least at first. Chronic asthma is marked by recurrent bronchospasm and airway inflammation, culminating in airway obstruction. The bronchi, not the alveoli, are affected by asthma.

Status Asthmaticus.

A severe acute attack of asthma that does not respond to normal treatment is known as status asthmaticus. A stimulus, such as an antigen that stimulates an allergic response, activates an inflammatory cascade that results in edema of the mucous membranes (swollen airway), contraction of smooth muscles (bronchospasm), increased mucus production (cough and blockage), and hyperinflation of the airways (decreased ventilation and shunting).

Air leak syndromes

Air leak syndromes can cause serious respiratory problems. Leaks can happen on their own or as a result of trauma (accidental, mechanical, or iatrogenic) or disease. The alveolar wall pulls away from the perivascular sheath when pressure rises inside the alveoli, and subsequent alveolar rupture allows air to follow the perivascular planes and flow into adjacent locations. Pneumothorax is defined as air in the pleural space causing a lung to collapse, and Barotrauma/volutrauma is defined as air in the interstitial space causing a lung to collapse (usually resolve over time).

Empyema and Pleural Effusion

Pleural effusion is a fluid accumulation in the pleural space caused by different diseases such as heart failure, tuberculosis, neoplasms, nephrotic syndrome, and viral respiratory infections. The fluid can be serous, bloody, or purulent (empyema), and it can be either transudative or exudative. The signs and symptoms of dyspnea range from moderate to severe, depending on the underlying disease.

Empyema is a type of pleural effusion in which a thick, purulent accumulation of pleural fluid forms as a result of bacterial pneumonia or severe chest trauma. Thoracentesis or thoracic surgery can cause empyema as a side effect. Acute sickness, fever, cold, pain, cough, and dyspnea are it's of the signs and symptoms.

Pulmonary fibrosis

Pulmonary fibrosis is a lung condition that causes the lining of the lungs to thicken due to scarring of the tissue. This thickness inhibits proper oxygen exchange from taking place. Although the exact etiology of pulmonary fibrosis is unknown, environmental pollutants like asbestos, infections, smoking and occupational exposure to wood or metal particles may all play a role.

Pulmonary Hypertension and Pulmonary Arterial Hypertension

Pulmonary arterial hypertension (PAH) is a progressive illness of the pulmonary arteries that can put patients' lives in jeopardy. It could be a combination of processes. The pulmonary vasculature usually adjusts quickly to accommodate the right ventricle's blood volume. When blood flow is increased, low resistance produces vasodilation and vice versa.

Primary (idiopathic) pulmonary hypertension and pulmonary arterial hypertension (PAH) are two types of pulmonary hypertension.

Identifying and treating any underlying cardiac or pulmonary disease, controlling symptoms, and preventing consequences are all goals of medical treatment for pulmonary arterial hypertension (PAH).

Respiratory Interventions and Procedures

Non-invasive Ventilation

- **Nasal Cannula:** A cannula for the nose can be used to supply supplemental oxygen to a patient, but it is only effective at flow rates of less than 6 L/min, as greater rates cause the nasal passages to dry out.
- **Non-Rebreather Mask:** that does not require rebreathing can be provided for patients who can breathe independently, to supply a higher oxygen concentration (60-90 percent).

Non-invasive positive pressure ventilators

Non-invasive positive pressure ventilators deliver air through a tight-fitting nose or face mask that is pressure cycled, eliminating the need for intubation and lowering the risk of hospital-acquired infection and mortality. It can be used to treat pulmonary edema and abrupt respiratory failure. CPAP (Continuous positive airway pressure), which provides a steady stream of pressurized air throughout both inspiration and expiration, and Bi-PAP (Bi-level positive airway pressure), which provides a steady stream of pressurized air as CPAP but senses inspiratory effort and increases pressure during inspiration, are the two types of non-invasive positive pressure ventilators.

Face Mask

It's critical to get the right fit and type of face mask (Ambu bag) for proper ventilation, oxygenation, and aspiration prevention.

Oxygen Delivery in High and Low Flows

At specified medium to high FIO_2, up to 100%, high flow oxygen delivery systems offer oxygen at flow rates higher than the patient's inspiratory flow rate. Low-flow oxygen delivery systems deliver 100 percent oxygen at lower flow rates than the patient's inspiratory flow rate, but the oxygen mixes with ambient air, causing the FIO_2 to fluctuate.

Airway Devices

TRACHEOSTOMY, OROPHARYNGEAL, AND NASOPHARYNGEAL TUBES Airways are utilized to provide a patent airway and make breathing easier.

Airway of the Laryngeal Mask.

The laryngeal-mask airway (LMA) is a type of intermediate airway that allows breathing but does not provide total respiratory control. The LMA is made up of an inflatable cuff (mask) and a tube that connects them. It can be used for a short time before tracheal intubation or when tracheal intubation is not possible.

Esophageal-Tracheal Combitube

The esophageal tracheal Combitube® (ETC) is a two-lumen intermediate airway that can be put into the trachea or the esophagus (91 percent of the time). The twin-lumen tube has a proximal cuff that seals the oropharynx, as well as a distal cuff that seals the distal tube.

Endotracheal Intubation is a form of a tracheal tube that is almost often introduced through the mouth (orotracheal) or nose (endotracheal) (nasotracheal). With respiratory failure, endotracheal intubation is frequently required to treat hypoxemia, hypercapnia, hypoventilation, and/or an obstructed airway. With a 10 mL syringe, examine tubes and connections for air leaks once they've been constructed.

Thoracentesis

To make a diagnosis, relieve pressure on the lung caused by pleural effusion, or administer drugs, a thoracentesis (aspiration of fluid or air from the pleural space) is performed.

Bronchoscopy

Bronchoscopy is a diagnostic procedure that uses a thin, flexible fiberoptic bronchoscope to examine the larynx, trachea, and bronchi. It can also be used to obtain biopsies, remove foreign substances or secretions, cure atelectasis, and excise lesions.

Thoracic Surgery is a type of surgery that is performed on the lungs.

Lung Volume Reduction is a condition in which the volume of the lungs is reduced Lung volume reduction surgery (LVRS) includes removing roughly 20-35 percent of non-functioning lung tissue to lower lung size and make the lungs perform more effectively. Adults with emphysematous COPD are the most typical candidates for this surgery.

Pneumonectomy. The surgical removal of one of the lungs is known as a pneumonectomy. There are two surgical procedures: basic, which involves removing only the lung, and extra pleural, which involves removing not only the lung but also a portion of the diaphragm and the pericardium on the affected side.

Lobectomy, and Other Procedures USED to Remove Partial Lung Tissue.

Lobectomy is a procedure that removes one or more lobes of the lung (there are two on the left and three on the right) and is used to treat lesions or trauma that affect only one lobe, such as tuberculosis, abscesses or cysts, cancer (usually non-small-cell in early stages), traumatic injury, or bronchiectasis. An open thoracotomy or a video-assisted thoracotomy is commonly used during surgery.

Pharmacology of the Respiratory System

Pharmacological Agents in the Management of Asthma

For asthma control, a variety of pharmacological medications are employed, some of which are long-acting to avoid attacks and others which are short-acting to provide relief during acute episodes. The following are the most common medications used in emergency situations. beta-adrenergic, anticholinergics, corticosteroids, methylprednisolone, methylxanthines, magnesium sulfate, heliox (helium-oxygen), and leukotriene inhibitors are some of the medications used to treat these conditions.

Pulmonary Pharmacology

Depending on the kind and severity of pulmonary disease, a variety of medicines are employed in pulmonary pharmacology. Opioid analgesics, neuromuscular blockers, human b-type natriuretic peptides, surfactants, alkalinizers, a pulmonary vasodilator (inhaled nitric oxide), methylxanthines, diuretics, nitrates, antibiotics, antimycobacterial, and antivirals are some of the medications used.

Chapter Six: **Endocrine System**

Pathophysiology of the Endocrine System

Types I and II Diabetes Mellitus

The most common metabolic condition is diabetes mellitus. Diabetes affects around 6% of Americans, although barely two-thirds are diagnosed.

- **Type I:** An immune-mediated condition in which the pancreatic beta cells are destroyed, resulting in inadequate insulin production. Insulin as needed to manage blood sugar, glucose monitoring 1-4 times daily, a carbohydrate-controlled diet, and exercise are all part of the treatment plan.
- **Type II:** Insulin resistance with an insulin secretion abnormality. Diet and exercise, glucose monitoring, and oral medications are all part of the treatment plan.

Ketoacidosis in Diabetes

Diabetic ketoacidosis is a type 1 diabetic complication caused by non-compliance with medication, stress, illness, or a lack of knowledge of having diabetes (this event often being the first time that diabetes is diagnosed). Potassium in cells shifts to the serum in any sort of acidosis. Ketone bodies cause ketoacidosis by lowering serum pH. Fluids, insulin, potassium, sodium, and magnesium, as well as electrolytes, are used to treat DKA.

HHNK

Hyperglycemic hyperosmolar nonketotic syndrome (HHNK) is a kind of diabetes that causes persistent hyperglycemia and osmotic diuresis in people who have never had diabetes or who have moderate type 2 diabetes. To maintain osmotic balance, fluid moves from intracellular to extracellular regions. Hypernatremia and increased osmolarity come from increased glucosuria and dehydration. Insulin drip with frequent (hourly) blood sugar monitoring, intravenous fluids and electrolytes, and correction of blood glucose and other labs are all used to treat ketoacidosis.

Acute Hypoglycemia

Pancreatic islet tumors or hyperplasia can cause acute hypoglycemia (hyperinsulinism). boosting insulin production or using insulin to manage diabetic Mellitus Treatment is based on the underlying cause and may include glucose/glucagon delivery, diazoxide (Hyperstat@) to limit insulin release, somatostatin (Sandostatin®) to reduce insulin production, and careful monitoring.

Diabetes Insipidus

A shortage of the antidiuretic hormone (ADH), also known as vasopressin, causes diabetes insipidus (DI). DI can occur as a result of head trauma, a primary brain tumor, meningitis, encephalitis, pituitary gland surgery or irradiation, or metastatic tumors. This differs to congenital nephrogenic diabetes insipidus, which has normal ADH generation but no response from the renal tubules. Hormonal (desmopressin) and nonhormonal medications are used to treat the condition (diuretics, vasopressin-releasing drugs, and prostaglandin inhibitors)

SIADH

(Syndrome of Inappropriate Antidiuretic Hormone Secretion) is caused by excessive secretion of antidiuretic hormone by the posterior pituitary gland. This causes the kidneys to reabsorb fluids, resulting in fluid retention, as well as a drop in sodium levels (dilutional hyponatremia), resulting in only concentrated urine being produced. Correction of fluid volume excess and electrolytes, as well as continuous urine output monitoring and seizure precautions, are all part of the treatment.

Addison's Disease (Chronic Adrenal Insufficiency)

Damage to the adrenal cortex can be caused by a variety of factors, including autoimmune disease or hereditary diseases, but it can also be caused by destructive lesions or neoplasms. The condition is life-threatening if not treated. Hormone replacement therapy with glucocorticoids (cortisol) and mineralocorticoids (aldosterone), which can be given orally or through monthly parenteral injections, is used to treat the condition. For women, androgen replacement therapy is sometimes suggested.

Acute Adrenal Insufficiency (Adrenal Crisis)

It is a condition in which the adrenal glands are severely underdeveloped. Acute adrenal insufficiency (adrenal crisis) is a life-threatening condition caused by an exacerbation of primary chronic adrenal insufficiency (Addison's disease), which is frequently triggered by sepsis, surgical stress, septicemia-related adrenal hemorrhage, anticoagulation complications, and cortisone withdrawal due to a reduced or inadequate dose to compensate for stress. IV fluids in high quantities, glucocorticoids, 50 percent dextrose if indicated (hypoglycemia), and mineralocorticoids may be required after intravenous solutions.

Hyperthyroidism

Excess thyroid hormone production (Graves' disease) from immunoglobulins supplying inappropriate thyroid gland stimulation causes hyperthyroidism (thyrotoxicosis). Thyroiditis and excessive thyroid medication are two other explanations. Treatment options include radioactive iodine to destroy the thyroid gland, antithyroid medicines (such as Propacil® or Tapazole® to block T4 to T3), and thyroid surgery if patients are unable to tolerate other therapies or have a significant goiter.

Thyrotoxic Storm

Thyrotoxic storm is a severe form of hyperthyroidism that manifests suddenly in persons who are untreated or inadequately treated for hyperthyroidism and is triggered by stress such as injury or surgery. It is lethal if not diagnosed and treated promptly. Controlling thyroid hormone production with antithyroid medications, inhibiting thyroid hormone release with iodine therapy (or lithium), controlling thyroid hormone peripheral activity with propranolol, fluid and electrolyte replacement, glucocorticoids like dexamethasone, cooling blankets, and treating arrhythmias as needed with antiarrhythmics and anticoagulants are all options for treatment.

Hypothyroidism

When the thyroid generates insufficient amounts of thyroid hormones, hypothyroidism develops. Myxedema can range in severity from minor to severe. Treatment involves replacing hormones with synthetic levothyroxine (Synthroid®) based on TSH levels, although this raises the body's oxygen demand, necessitating careful cardiac monitoring early on to avoid myocardial infarction while achieving euthyroid (normal) levels.

Cushing's Syndrome and Cushing's Disease

When cortisol levels rise, Cushing syndrome develops. This is most usually caused by prednisone steroid therapy. Causes of Endogenous include a pituitary adenoma that produces excessive quantities of adrenocorticotropic hormone (ACTH) and generates elevated cortisol (Cushing's disease) or an adrenal gland primary tumor that causes increased cortisol output.

Hyperparathyroidism

When the parathyroid hormone is overproduced, hyperparathyroidism develops (PTH). The normal range is between 10 and 55 pg/mL. The most prevalent symptom of hyperparathyroidism is hypercalcemia (total calcium >10.4 mg/dL).

Hypoparathyroidism

PTH deficiency causes hypoparathyroidism. This occurs more frequently in women and is mainly caused by an accident during thyroid/neck surgery, radioactive iodine treatment for hyperthyroidism, radiation, or autoimmune reasons.

Pharmacology of the Endocrine System

Hypoglycemic Agents (Oral)

Oral hypoglycemic medicines are anti-diabetic medications that are commonly used to treat Type 2 diabetes. Sulfonylureas, biguanides, meglitinides, competitive inhibitors of alpha-glucosidases (found in the intestinal brush border), and thiazolidinediones are the five most common types of oral hypoglycemic medicines. Recently, two new kinds of oral hypoglycemics, DPP-4 inhibitors, and SGLT2 inhibitors were launched both of which are beneficial when used in conjunction with dietary and activity improvements.

Insulin is Used in the Treatment of Glycemic Diseases.

Insulin comes in a variety of forms, each having a different action time. Insulin is utilized to metabolize glucose in people who don't have insulin-producing pancreases. To maintain glucose control, people may need to take a mixture of insulins (short and long-acting).

Chapter Seven:
Immune System

Pathophysiology of the Immune System

Deficiencies in the Immune System

Primary immunodeficiency illnesses are a group of diseases that affect the immune system. These are genetic or inherited illnesses in which the immune system of the body fails to operate properly. Low amounts of antibodies, flaws in antibodies, or deficiencies in immune system cells can all cause these problems (T-cells, B-cells). Immunoglobulin replacement is commonly given to patients with immune deficiency illnesses. Recurrent infections may also necessitate the use of long-term antibiotics. Patients should be taught to wash their hands regularly, thoroughly cook their foods, avoid large crowds, and use other infection-prevention practices.

Congenital Immunodeficiencies

The following are examples of congenital immunodeficiencies:

- Variable immunodeficiency syndrome
- Agammaglobulinemia congenital (Bruton's, x-linked)

- Selective IgA deficiency
- Wiskott-Aldrich syndrome.

Compensate for Deficiencies

All elements of the complement pathway are deficient, including the following:

- C1 (q, r, s), C2, and C4 are examples of classic deficits.
- Deficiency in C3 and alternative complements
- Deficiency of the membrane attack complex (MAC) is also known as terminal complement deficiency.

Autoimmune System Disorders

Allergic interstitial/tubulointerstitial nephritis is a type of interstitial/tubulointerstitial nephritis that affects the kidneys

- Eosinophilic esophagitis
- Churg-Strauss syndrome (AKA eosinophilic granulomatosis with polyangiitis).

Neutropenia

Neutropenia is defined as a polymorphonuclear neutrophil count of 500 or fewer per milliliter of blood. Chronic neutropenia is a condition in which the number of neutrophils in the blood is reduced to zero for three months or more. A decrease in white blood cell production can cause neutropenia.

Leukopenia

A decrease in white blood cells is known as leukopenia. The term "neutropenia" is commonly used interchangeably with "leukopenia," which refers to a low number of neutrophils. In the treatment of leukopenia, supportive care is used, as well as rigorous treatment of any infections that may arise. Hematopoietic growth agents may also be used to boost neutrophil production.

Lymphedema

Lymphedema is caused by edema that has gone untreated or is incurable. Swelling and collected fluids within the tissue characterize this chronic disease. Lymphatic drainage failure, insufficient lymph transport capacity, excessive lymph production, or a combination of these factors cause this buildup.

HIV/AIDS

AIDS is a disease caused by the human immunodeficiency virus (HIV). When the following conditions are met, AIDS is diagnosed:

- Infection with HIV.
- Is your CD4 count less than 200 cells per millimeter?
- AIDS-defining conditions include opportunistic infections (cytomegalovirus, TB), wasting syndrome, neoplasms (Kaposi sarcoma), and the AIDS dementia complex.

Because there are so many different AIDS-defining diseases, the patient may exhibit a variety of symptoms depending on the diagnosis. Highly active antiretroviral therapy (HAART), which involves the administration of three or more medications at the same time, attempts to cure or manage opportunistic infections while also controlling underlying HIV infection.

Chapter Eight: **Hematology**

Pathophysiology of Hematology

Anemia

Anemia is a condition in which the body's oxygen supply is insufficient due to a lack of red blood cells. The body will try to compensate for the lower oxygen supply to the organs by boosting cardiac output and shifting blood to the brain and heart.

Sickle Cell Disease

Sickle cell disease is a chromosome 11 recessive genetic illness that causes hemoglobin to be faulty, causing sickle-shaped and inflexible red blood cells (RBCs) to accumulate in narrow capillaries and cause painful obstruction. Normal RBCs can live for 120 days, but sickled cells can only live for 10 to 20 days, putting a strain on the bone marrow, which can't create enough blood, resulting in severe anemia.

Vera Polycythemia

Polycythemia vera is a disorder in which the bone marrow produces abnormally large amounts of blood cells. Erythrocytes (red blood cells) are the most affected cells.

Von Willebrand Disease

Von Willebrand disease is a group of congenital bleeding disorders caused by a deficiency or lack of von Willebrand factor (vWF), a glycoprotein synthesized, stored, and secreted by vascular endothelial cells. It affects 1-2 percent of the population. Type I, Type II, and Type III are the three types.

Disseminated Intravascular Coagulation

Trauma, congenital heart disease, necrotizing enterocolitis, sepsis, and severe viral infections can all produce disseminated intravascular coagulation (DIC) (consumption coagulopathy), which is a secondary condition. Through a complex chain of events, DIC causes both coagulation and bleeding.

Thrombocytopenia

A lack of circulating platelets in the blood is known as thrombocytopenia. It can be caused by a decrease in platelet synthesis from the bone marrow or an increase in platelet breakdown. The usage of heparin might also result in thrombocytopenia.

ITP

Idiopathic thrombocytopenic purpura (ITP) is an autoimmune illness that produces an immune reaction to platelets, resulting in low platelet levels. ITP primarily affects children and young women; however, it can strike anyone at any age. The acute form primarily affects youngsters, while the chronic form primarily affects adults.

HITTS

Heparin-induced thrombocytopenia and thrombosis syndrome (HITTS) is a thrombocytopenia and thrombosis syndrome that arises in people who are using heparin for anticoagulation. Type I and Type II are the two types.

Coagulopathy Induced by Reopro

By suppressing platelet aggregation, ReoPro® (abciximab) is used to reduce myocardial ischemia in people having percutaneous cardiac intervention. It increases the effectiveness of anticoagulants when used with aspirin and/or weight-adjusted low-dose heparin.

Interventions and Procedures in Hematology

Components of Transfusion

Packed red blood cells, platelet concentrates, fresh frozen plasma (FFP), and cryoprecipitate are all popular blood components used in transfusions.

Autotransfusion

Autotransfusion (autologous blood transfusion) is the collection and re-infusion of a patient's blood. If another donor's blood is unavailable, this is life-saving. Blood is generally taken from a bodily cavity in trauma instances, such as the pleural (hemothorax with 21,500 mL blood) or peritoneal space (rare).

Plasmapheresis

Plasmapheresis involves the removal of whole blood from the body, the addition of an anticoagulant, the separation of cellular components from plasma (which is removed), and the suspension of cellular components in saline, albumin (the most frequent), or another plasma substitute.

Transfusion of Exchange

To remove sickled blood for sickle cell anemia or to eliminate toxins, exchange transfusions, replace a person's blood with donor blood. The swap may be entire or partial. Typically, an automated machine is employed, with a period on the machine ranging from 1 to 4 hours.

Depletion of Leukocyte

Transfusions of red blood cells and platelets frequently contain leukocytes, which the immune system of the patient receiving the transfusion recognizes as alien. This can have negative consequences, especially in immunocompromised patients. Various techniques, including filtration, are used to deplete leukocytes.

Administration of Transfusion

The nurse should get the patient's transfusion history as well as a consent document before administering any blood component. The patient's blood must be typed and crossmatched, and an IV must be in place for administration. A normal catheter is 18 gauge, although a 22-gauge catheter can be used at a slower rate.

Conservation of Blood

Blood conservation methods include minimizing blood loss during surgical procedures, lowering the threshold for getting transfusions, maintaining an adequate hematocrit, and ensuring optimal tissue oxygenation.

Protocol for Massive Transfusion

A massive transfusion protocol (MTP) is a proactive defined approach that is utilized during an uncontrolled hemorrhage to ensure appropriate management of enormous blood loss and enhance patient outcomes.

Complications Related to Transfusion

There are several transfusion-related problems, which is why transfusions are only administered when necessary. Infection, transfusion-related acute lung injury (TRALI), graft vs. host illness, post-transfusion purpura, transfusion-related immunosuppression, and hypothermia are all possible complications.

Hematologic Pharmacology

Anticoagulants

Antithrombin activators, direct thrombin inhibitors, antithrombin (AT), and warfarin are all common anticoagulants used at home and in hospitals.

Heparin

Heparin is an anticoagulant made from the mucosa of the pig's intestinal mucosa and the lung of the pig. Heparin's mode of action is to bind to the endothelial cell membrane's surface. Antithrombin III, a plasma protease inhibitor, is required for heparin's function. Thrombin and other anti-clotting proteases are inhibited by Antithrombin III. Heparin-binding also changes the shape of the antithrombin III inhibitor, resulting in increased antithrombin-protease complex formation activity.

Warfarin

Warfarin is an antithrombotic drug that reduces the risk of embolism in humans by causing a prothrombin deficit in the plasma. This substance affects the liver to produce fewer of the proteins required for blood coagulation. Warfarin has a high bioavailability since it is 99 percent linked to albumin in the plasma. Prothrombin, factor VII, factor IX, factor X, and protein C are all involved in warfarin's mechanism of action. The g-carboxylation of glutamate residues in the aforementioned variables is inhibited by warfarin. Vitamin K is also involved in the action of warfarin.

Thrombolytics

Thrombolytics are medications that dissolve blood clots in the event of a heart attack, ischemic stroke, DVT, or pulmonary embolism. To increase the anticoagulation effect, thrombolytics can be used in conjunction with heparin or low-weight heparin. Alteplase tissue-type plasminogen activator (t-PA) (Activase@®), Anistreplase (Eminase®), Reteplase (Retavase®), Streptokinase (Streptase®), Tenecteplase (TNKase®), Streptokinase (Streptase®), Tenecteplase (TNKase®).

Chapter Nine: **Nervous System**

Pathophysiology of the Nervous System

Encephalopathies

Hypertensive encephalopathy with cerebral edema hypertensive. A hypertensive crisis can lead to hypertensive encephalopathy. The brain adjusts to greater pressures to regulate blood flow in chronic hypertension, but in a hypertensive emergency, the blood-brain barrier is overcome, and the capillaries leak fluid into the tissue, causing vasodilation and cerebral edema.

Encephalopathy In Hypoxic Conditions

When the oxygen supply to the brain is reduced, cerebral hypoxia (hypoxic encephalopathy) ensues. The brain adapts for mild hypoxia by boosting cerebral blood flow, but it can only double in volume and is unable to compensate for severe hypoxia. Hypoxia can be caused by a lack of oxygen in the environment, a lack of exchange at the alveolar level of the lungs, or a lack of blood flow to the brain.

Metabolic Encephalopathy

Damage to the brain caused by a disruption in metabolism, especially hepatic failure to eliminate poisons from the blood, is known as metabolic encephalopathy (hepatic encephalopathy). There could be a reduction in cerebral blood flow, edema, or an increase in intracranial pressure.

Encephalopathy Infectious

Infectious encephalopathy is a broad term that encompasses encephalopathies caused by a variety of bacteria, viruses, or prions. All infections cause changed brain function, which causes changes in consciousness and personality, as well as cognitive impairment and lethargy.

Cerebral Aneurysms

The majority of cerebral aneurysms (the weakening and dilatation of a cerebral artery) are congenital (90 percent), whereas the remaining 10% are caused by direct trauma or infection. Aneurysms in the Circle of Willis near the base of the brain are generally 2-7 mm in diameter.

Malformation of the Arteriovenous System

Arteriovenous malformation (AVM) is a congenital brain disorder characterized by a tangle of dilated arteries and veins with no capillary bed. AVMs can appear anywhere in the brain and may not cause any symptoms. One or more cerebral arteries "feed" the AVM, which expands over time, shunting more blood via the AVM.

Intraventricular/Intracranial Hemorrhage

Epidural And Subdural. Bleeding between the dura and the skull forces the brain downward and inward, causing epidural hemorrhage. Because arterial tears are the most common source of hemorrhage, bleeding is generally fast, resulting in severe neurological impairments and respiratory collapse.

Subdural hemorrhage is bleeding between the dura and the cerebrum, which is caused by tears in the subdural space's cortical veins. It takes longer to develop than epidural hemorrhage and can lead to a subdural hematoma.

Subarachnoid

SAH can arise as a result of trauma, however, it is more commonly caused by the rupture of a vascular aneurysm or an arteriovenous malformation (AVM).

Communicating and Noncommunicating Hydrocephalus

Cerebrospinal fluid is produced and circulated by the ventricular system (CSF). There are two types of hydrocephalus:

- In Communicating, CSF moves between the ventricles (communicates), but it is not absorbed in the subarachnoid region (arachnoid villi).
- In non-communicating, CSF is occluded (non-communicating) between the ventricles, with the obstruction most commonly caused by stenosis of the Sylvius aqueduct.

Neurologic Infectious Disease

Meningitis Caused by Bacteria

Streptococcus pneumonia and Neisseria meningitides are just two bacteria that can cause bacterial meningitis. Bacteria can reach the CNS through a variety of routes, including a distant infection, surgical wounds, invasive devices, nasal colonization, and penetrating trauma. Inflammation, exudates, WBC buildup, and brain tissue destruction with hyperemia and edema are all part of the infective process. Purulent exudate coats the brain, infiltrating and blocking the ventricles, restricting CSF and raising intracranial pressure.

Meningitis Caused by Fungus

Meningitis caused by fungus is the least prevalent type of meningitis. When a fungal organism reaches the subarachnoid space, cerebral spinal fluid, or meninges, it causes meningitis. Candida albicans and Cryptococcus neoformans are the most prevalent organisms that cause fungal meningitis.

Infections that can Affect the Neurological System

- Arboviral infections are transmitted from an animal host to an arthropod (usually a mosquito or tick) and then to humans, who are usually dead-end hosts.
- Viral meningitis is less severe than bacterial meningitis and normally resolves within 7 to 10 days.
- Herpes simplex virus: Herpes simplex virus can infect the neurological system and cause herpes simplex encephalitis, which is fatal.
- Inflammation in the CNS can disrupt neuronal processes and cause HIV.

Disorders of the Neuromuscular System

Multiple Sclerosis

Multiple sclerosis is a CNS autoimmune illness in which the myelin sheath around nerves is destroyed and replaced by scar tissue, preventing nerve impulses from being transmitted.

ALS

Amyotrophic lateral sclerosis (ALS) is a progressive degenerative disease of the upper and lower motor neurons that causes dysphagia, cramping, muscular atrophy, and respiratory dysfunction. It causes spasticity, hyperreflexia, muscle weakness, and paralysis. ALS can be sporadic or run in families (rare). Your speech may grow monotonous.

Parkinson's Disease

Parkinson's disease (PD) is a motor system condition characterized by the loss of dopamine-producing brain cells.

Guillain-Barre Syndrome

Guillain-Barré syndrome (GBS) is a myelinated motor peripheral nerve system autoimmune illness that causes ascending and descending paralysis. GBS is frequently caused by a viral infection, however, it can also be idiopathic.

Dystrophy of the Muscutum

Muscular dystrophies are hereditary illnesses that cause muscle fiber degradation, skeletal muscle weakening and atrophy, and loss of movement. The most frequent and severe kind of muscular dystrophy is pseudohypertrophic (Duchenne) muscular dystrophy.

Palsy of the Cerebral Nervous System

Cerebral palsy (CP) is a non-progressive motor dysfunction caused by CNS impairment caused by congenital, hypoxic, or traumatic injury before, during, or within the first two years of life. Visual problems, verbal difficulties, convulsions, and mental retardation are all possible symptoms. Spastic, dyskinetic, ataxic, and mixed motor dysfunction are the four forms of motor dysfunction.

Myasthenia Gravis

Myasthenia gravis is an autoimmune disease that causes sporadic, increasing weakening of striated (skeletal) muscles due to poor nerve impulse transmission. Myasthenia gravis often affects muscles controlled by the cranial nerves, but it can affect any muscle group. Thymomas are found in a large number of people.

Seizure Disorders

Partial Seizure

Electrical discharges to a limited portion of the cerebral cortex, such as the frontals, temporal, or parietal lobes, generate partial seizures with seizure features that are related to the area of involvement. They can start in a focal point and spread out, and they're commonly preceded by an aura. Simple partial (aversive and sylvan), special sensory, and complex sensory are all included (psychomotor).

Generalized Seizures

Generalized seizures do not have a focal onset and appear to affect both hemispheres, with loss of consciousness and no previous aura. It contains tonic-clonic (grand mal) and the absence of tonic-clonic (grand mal) (petit mal).

Epilepsy. A history of seizure activity, as well as supportive EEG data, are used to diagnose epilepsy. Individualized care is provided. Milder effects usually fade away with time or dose adjustments. Toxic effects might vary greatly based on the medication and the length of time it has been used, so careful monitoring is required.

Epilepticus status. Generalized tonic-clonic seizures, also known as status epilepticus (SE), are characterized by a sequence of seizures with insufficient time between them for regaining consciousness. Exhaustion, respiratory failure with hypoxemia and hypercapnia, heart failure, and mortality might result from the continual assault and periods of apnea.

Brain Tumors

Adults might get any sort of brain tumor. Brain tumors can be either primary (originating in the brain) or secondary (resulting from metastasis). Astrocytoma, glioblastoma, brain stem glioma, craniopharyngioma, meningioma, ganglioglioma, medulloblastoma, oligodendroglioma, and optical nerve glioma are some of the cancers that fall under this category.

Strokes

- **Strokes of the hemorrhagic system.** Hemorrhagic strokes account for roughly 20% of all strokes and are caused by a ruptured cerebral artery, which results in a shortage of oxygen and nutrients as well as edema, which causes extensive pressure and damage. Intracerebral aneurysms, intracranial aneurysms, arteriovenous malformations, and subarachnoid hemorrhage are all examples.
- **Strokes of ischemia.** Strokes (brain attacks, cerebrovascular accidents) occur when blood flow to a part of the brain is interrupted. Ischemic and hemorrhagic are the two most common kinds. Ischemic stroke affects about 80% of people, originating from a blockage in a brain artery.
- **TIA.** Small clots induce transient ischemic attacks (TIAs), which are comparable but less severe.

Brain Death

While each state has its laws describing the legal definition of brain death, most of them include something like this: If a person has "maintained irreversible cessation of circulatory and respiratory activities; or has sustained irreversible cessation of all functions of the entire brain, including the brain stem," they have brain death.

Delirium

Delirium is a state of consciousness that is sudden, abrupt, and variable. Drugs, infections, hypoxia, trauma, dementia, depression, visual and hearing loss, and surgery can all cause delirium. Malnutrition, drunkenness, untreated pain, fluid/electrolyte imbalance Delirium, if left untreated, dramatically raises the chance of death.

Agitation

In severely ill patients, agitation is a common occurrence. Drug or alcohol withdrawal, sleep deprivation, hypoxemia, electrolyte or metabolic imbalance, anxiety, pain, and bad drug reactions are among the factors that can lead to agitation. Agitation can be a symptom of delirium as well.

Dementia

Dementia is a chronic illness in which memory and function are gradually and irreversibly lost. A nurse may meet a variety of dementias, including:

- Creutzfeldt-Jakob disease
- Dementia with Lewy Bodies
- Frontotemporal dementia
- Dementia with a mix of symptoms.
- Hydrocephalus with normal pressure.
- Dementia caused by Parkinson's disease.
- Vascular dementia

Interventions and Procedures in Neurology

Clipping for Aneurysm Treatment

The risk of rebleeding, which is 4 percent in the first 24 hours and 1-2 percent each day for the next month, necessitates surgical clipping of a burst or big, unstable aneurysm. In most cases, surgical repair can be completed in less than 48 hours. Clipping can be done as a preventative measure to avoid rupture. The aneurysm is clipped to keep it from rupturing and obstructing circulation. To access the site of the aneurysm, a craniotomy and a brain incision are usually performed.

Embolization for Aneurysm or AVM Treatment

Embolization is a minimally invasive procedure that is used to treat aneurysms and AVMs as an alternative to cutting. Different forms of embolization exist, however they all rely on fluoroscopy and percutaneous transfemoral catheterization. The catheter is guided to the damaged area via the femoral and carotid arteries.

Surgical removal of an AVM

Both embolization and radiation treatments have the possibility of the aberrant vessels recurring, hence surgical removal of AVMs is the ultimate treatment for AVMs. Large AVMs may necessitate the use of two or more operations. Because the AVM is usually surrounded by non-functioning brain tissue, it can remove the AVM without damaging the brain tissue.

Craniotomy Patients' Postoperative Care

The patient must be closely monitored in the post-operative period following a craniotomy for any problems or changes in condition:

Burr Hoes

Burr holes are small holes drilled through the skull to relieve elevated intracranial pressure (such as from a subdural, epidural, or hydrocephalus hematoma), drain blood, or remove foreign items. Burr holes can also be utilized as access sites for brain surgeries that are less invasive, such as removing a brain tumor.

Interventions in the Neuro-Endovascular System

Coiling

Coiling is a minimally invasive treatment for treating aneurysms in the brain. In the femoral area, a catheter is placed and progressed to the aneurysm. Then a microcatheter with a coil attached is inserted into the aneurysm and fed through the catheter until the coil fills the aneurysm. The catheter is withdrawn after the coil is split with an electrical current. More than one coil may be required in some circumstances.

Thrombectomy

A thrombectomy is a technique that removes an endovascular clot. Various approaches may be utilized, but often, a catheter is introduced into the femoral vein and advanced to the clot, where it is suctioned, mechanically broken up, and the pieces removed, or a helical thrombectomy device is wrapped around the clot and removed. Thrombectomy is a procedure that restores blood flow after a stroke or removes clots in the arms or legs.

Pharmacology of the Nervous System

Anticonvulsants

Carbamazepine (Tegretol®), Clonazepam (Klonopin®), Ethosuximide (Zarontin®), Felbamate (Felbatol®), Fosphenytoin (Cerebyx®), Fosphenytoin (Cerebyx®), Gabapentin (Neurontin®), Lamotrigine (Lamictal®), Levetiracetam (Keppra®), Oxcarbazepine (Trileptal®), Phenobarbital (Luminal®), Phenytoin (Dilantin®), Primidone (Mysoline®), Tiagabine (Gabitril®), Topiramate (Topamax®), Valproate/Valproic acid (Depakote®, Depakene®), and Zonisamide (Zonegran®, Excegran®).

Hypertonic Saline Solution

Hypertonic saline solution (HSS) has a sodium content of more than 0.9 percent (NS) and is used to treat traumatic brain injury and relieve intracranial pressure/cerebral edema.

Mannitol

Mannitol is an osmotic diuretic that decreases intracranial pressure and brain mass after traumatic brain injury by increasing salt and water excretion. Mannitol can also be used to shrink the cells that make up the blood-brain barrier, allowing other drugs to pass through.

Chapter Ten:
Gastrointestinal Tract

Pathophysiology of the Gastrointestinal Tract

Peritonitis

Peritonitis (peritoneal inflammation) can be primary (caused by a blood or lymph infection) or secondary (caused by perforation or trauma to the gastrointestinal system). Perforated bowel, ruptured appendix, abdominal trauma, abdominal surgery, peritoneal dialysis or chemotherapy, or sterile fluid leakage into the peritoneum are all common causes. Intravenous fluids and electrolytes, broad-spectrum antibiotics, and, if necessary, laparoscopy are used to discover the source of peritonitis and repair it.

Appendicitis

Appendicitis is an inflammation of the appendix caused by secretions building up and finally perforating the appendix due to luminal blockage and pressure within the lumen. The fact that the exact position of the appendix varies from patient to patient might make diagnosis challenging. Appendectomy, laparoscopy, or open surgery are all options for treatment.

Cholecystitis

Cholecystitis can cause bile duct obstruction due to calculi, as well as pancreatitis due to pancreatic duct obstruction. Fever, leukocytosis, right upper quadrant stomach pain, and gallbladder inflammation are all symptoms of acute cholecystitis.

Antibiotics for sepsis/ascending cholangitis, antispasmodic agents (glycopyrrolate) for biliary colic and vomiting, analgesics (note that opioids cause increased sphincter of Oddi pressure), antiemetics, and surgical consultation for possible laparoscopic or open cholecystectomy are all options for treatment.

Nonerosive Gastritis vs. Erosive Gastritis

Gastritis is an inflammation of the stomach's epithelium or endothelium. The following are examples of different types:

- Erosive: Alcohol, NSAIDs, sickness, portal hypertension, and/or stress are the most common causes.
- Helicobacter pylori infection or pernicious anemia are the most common causes of non-erosive gastritis.

Gastroenteritis Viral. gastroenteritis nausea is a symptom of viral gastroenteritis (also known as stomach flu). Vomiting, abdominal cramps, watery (perhaps bloody) diarrhea, headache, muscle aches, and fever are all symptoms to look out for. The fecal-oral pathway is used to disseminate viral gastroenteritis. Norovirus and rotavirus are two common causes.

Bacterial Gastroenteritis. Cramping and nausea are common symptoms of bacterial gastroenteritis. as well as severe diarrhea Enterotoxins, which stick to the mucosa of the intestines, cause gastroenteritis in some bacteria, while exotoxins, which remain in infected food, cause gastroenteritis in others. Some bacteria directly infect the mucosa of the intestine. Bacterial gastroenteritis is a type of gastroenteritis caused by Salmonella, Campylobacters, Shigella species, and Escherichia coli.

Parasitic Gastroenteritis. Infection with the protozoa (one-celled pathogens) Giardia intestinalis and Cryptosporidium parvum is the most common cause of parasitic gastroenteritis.

Constipation Impaction

Constipation is defined as a condition in which a person's bowel motions are less frequent than normal, or when hard, tiny stool is excreted fewer than three times per week.

Fecal impaction occurs when a hard stool slides into the rectum and forms a huge, thick, immovable mass that can't be evacuated even with straining, which is most commonly caused by chronic constipation.

Causes Of Constipation and Medical Procedures to Evaluate Them

Medical techniques to determine the reason for constipation should be preceded by a thorough medical history, as this can assist define the type and guide the diagnostic procedures used. Physical examination, blood tests, abdominal x-ray, barium enema, colonic transit, defecography, anorectal manometry, colonic motility, or colonoscope are examples of medical diagnostic methods.

Bowel Obstructions

Bowel blockage occurs when the flow of intestinal contents is obstructed mechanically due to a constriction of the lumen, occlusion of the lumen, adhesion formation, or a lack of muscular contractions (paralytic ileus).

Bowel Infarctions

Ischemia of the intestines caused by a severely reduced blood supply is known as bowel infarction. It can be caused by a variety of disorders, including strangulated bowel or occlusion of the mesentery's arteries, and it can also occur as a result of untreated intestinal obstruction.

Perforation of the Intestinal System

A partial or full tear in the intestinal wall is known as intestinal perforation. intestine contents oozing into the peritoneum Trauma, NSAIDs (elderly, diverticulitis patients), acute appendicitis, PUD, iatrogenic (laparoscopy, endoscopy, colonoscopy, radiation), bacterial infections, IBS, and consumption of poisonous substances (acids) or foreign things are some of the causes (toothpicks).

Reflux of the Gastroesophageal System

When the lower esophageal sphincter fails to seal properly, the contents of the stomach can back up into the esophagus, causing gastroesophageal reflux (GER). The acid-containing contents of the stomach may reflux into the esophagus, irritating the esophageal lining. The lining of the esophagus can be damaged over time. Barrett's esophagus may develop in certain patients as a result of this.

Peptic Ulcer Disease

Peptic ulcer disease (PUD) affects both the duodenum and the stomach. They might be primary (typically duodenal) or secondary (usually esophageal) (usually gastric). H. pylori infections are the most common cause of gastric ulcers (80%), but aspirin and NSAIDs can also cause them. H. pylori cause chronic inflammation and ulcerations of the gastric mucosa and are spread via the fecal-oral route or contaminated water.

Inflammatory Bowel Disease

Ulcerative Colitis

Ulcerative colitis is a condition in which the mucosa of the colon and rectum becomes inflamed, resulting in ulcers in the places where the inflammation has damaged cells.

Crohn's Disease

Crohn's disease is characterized by gastrointestinal (GI) system inflammation. With aphthous ulcerations evolving to linear and irregular-shaped ulcerations, inflammation is transmural (frequently leading to intestinal stenosis and fistulas), localized, and discontinuous. There may be granulomas present. The terminal ileum and cecum are common sites of inflammation.

Diverticular Disease

Diverticular disease is characterized by the presence of diverticula (saclike pouching of the bowel lining that expands through a defect in the muscular layer) anywhere throughout the GI tract. Acute diverticulitis occurs when the diverticula become inflamed as a result of food or germs being retained within the diverticula, which affects about 20% of people with diverticular disease. Abscess, blockage, perforation, hemorrhage, or a fistula are all possible outcomes.

Acute Gastrointestinal Hemorrhage

A hemorrhage in the upper or lower gastrointestinal tract is known as a GI hemorrhage. Gastric and duodenal ulcers, which are commonly caused by stress, NSAIDs, or infection with Helicobacter pylori, are the leading cause of GI hemorrhage (50-70 percent).

Hernias

Hernias are protrusions into or through the abdominal wall that can happen to both children and adults. Fat, tissue, or bowel can all be seen in hernias. Direct inguinal hernias, indirect inguinal hernias, femoral hernias, umbilical hernias, and incisional hernias are some of the several forms. Obesity or wound infections are the most common causes, and they can lead to incarceration.

Cirrhosis in the Liver

- **Compensated.** Compensated Cirrhosis is a chronic hepatic condition in which normal liver tissue is replaced by fibrotic tissue, causing the liver function to be impaired. There are three forms of alcoholic liver disease: alcoholic, post-necrotic, and biliary.
- **Decompensated.** Decompensated cirrhosis develops when the liver's ability to manufacture proteins, clotting factors, and other chemicals are compromised, resulting in portal hypertension.

Fulminant Hepatitis

Fulminant hepatitis is a severe acute liver infection that can cause hepatic necrosis, encephalopathy, and death in as little as two weeks. According to the length of time from jaundice to encephalopathy, fulminant hepatitis can be split into three stages:

- Hyperacute liver failure is defined as a period between 0 and 7 days.
- Acute liver failure lasts 7 to 28 days.
- Subacute liver failure lasts 28 to 72 days.

Hypertension of the Portal System

When blood flow is impeded in the portal venous system, blood pressure rises, preventing the liver from filtering blood and triggering the formation of collateral blood capillaries that return unfiltered blood to the systemic circulation.

Variations in the Esophageal System

Esophageal varices are dilated, tortuous veins in the esophagus's submucosa (usually the distal portion). They are a complication of liver cirrhosis in which obstruction of the portal vein causes an increase in collateral veins and a decrease in liver circulation, raising the pressure in the collateral arteries.

Hepatic Coma

When the liver's ability to eliminate ammonia and other poisons from the bloodstream is compromised, hepatic coma or hepatic encephalopathy develops. Patients with severe liver disease, most often cirrhosis of the liver, are more likely to develop hepatic encephalopathy.

Biliary Atresia

Biliary atresia is a life-threatening disorder that affects children and is caused by an unknown factor. Biliary atresia develops when the bile ducts (either inside or outside the liver) become inflamed, resulting in duct damage and bile flow obstruction.

Acute Pancreatitis

In 90% of cases, acute pancreatitis is linked to persistent drinking or cholelithiasis, but the cause may be unclear. It can also be brought on by several medications (tetracycline, thiazides, acetaminophen, and oral contraceptives).

Interventions and Procedures for the Gastrointestinal Tract

Levin Tubes, NG Tubes, and Sump Tubes

Plastic or vinyl tubes are introduced through the nose, down the esophagus, and into the stomach. To prevent a vacuum from building with heavy suction, sump tubes are radiopaque and have a vent lumen. Levin tubes do not have a vent lumen and are only utilized when suction is low. NG tubes are used to drain gastric secretions, sample them, or get access to the stomach and upper GI tract. They're utilized for lavage following a medicine overdose, decompression, and medication or fluid instillation. NG tubes should not be used if there is a proximal obstruction to the stomach or if there is a gastric pathology, such as hemorrhage.

PEG Tube

PEG involves intubating the esophagus with an endoscope and inserting a sheathed needle with a guidewire through the abdomen and stomach wall so that a catheter can be fed down the esophagus, snared, and drawn out through the orifice where the needle was entered and secured.

Drains

The following are the various types of drains that a patient could have, along with nursing considerations: Simple drains, Penrose drains, sump drains, percutaneous drainage catheters, and closed drainage systems (Jackson-Pratt® and Hemovac®) are some of the options available.

Parental Support as Well as Enteral Support

Enteral nutrition is a way of feeding a patient through a tube, which can be inserted in the nose (a nasogastric tube), the stomach (a percutaneous endoscopic gastrostomy [PEG] tube), or the small bowel (a percutaneous endoscopic gastrostomy [PEG] tube) (a percutaneous endoscopic jejunal [J] tube).

Parenteral nutrition (also known as total parenteral nutrition [TPN]) is a type of nutrition delivery that bypasses the digestive system entirely by using an intravenous line. Although enteral nutrition is preferred, when a patient's gastrointestinal tract is compromised, parenteral nourishment is the sole option.

Whipple in Gastrointestinal Surgery.

The Whipple (pancreaticoduodenectomy) procedure removes the head of the pancreas, the gallbladder, a piece of the bile duct, the duodenum, and sometimes the distal region of the stomach through surgery.

Esophagogastrectomy and esophagectomy. The removal of all or part of the esophagus, with the distal end restored to the stomach or an intestinal graft utilized to replace the excised segment of the esophagus, is known as esophagectomy. The distal segment of the esophagus, lymph nodes, and the upper region of the stomach is removed during an esophagogastrectomy, following which the remaining esophagus and stomach are reattached.

Gastrointestinal surgery in bariatric patients. Bariatric surgery is used to help morbidly obese people lose weight (100 pounds over normal weight or BMI of 35-40). Surgery is performed to limit calorie intake and/or prevent calorie absorption. Banding, sleeve gastrectomy, Roux-en-Y, and gastric ballooning are open surgical or laparoscopic procedures that implant a balloon in the stomach and fill it with fluids to reduce stomach capacity; this is mostly performed in Europe.

Fecal Management Systems in Indwelling

Incontinent clients with loose or watery feces are given indwelling fecal management systems to prevent skin breakdown, discomfort, odor, and wound infection, as well as to restrict the spread of germs like Clostridium difficile in bedridden or immobile clients. A silicone catheter, a silicone retention balloon at the end of the catheter, a 45-mL syringe, and charcoal filter collection bags are typical components of a management system.

Pharmacology of the Gastrointestinal Tract

Antagonists to Histamine Receptor

Histamine (H) receptor antagonists (really reverse agonists) are used to treat heartburn and GERD caused by too much stomach acid. They reduce acid production by blocking histamine 2 (H:) (parietal) cell receptors in the stomach. Cimetidine (Tagamet®), ranitidine (Zantac®), famotidine (Pepcid®), and nizatidine (Axid®) are all common H2 antagonists.

Antacids

Antacids are drugs that work by raising the pH of the stomach and neutralizing the acids present. They're widely used to alleviate indigestion and heartburn. Aluminum hydroxide (Amphojel®), magnesium hydroxide (Milk of Magnesia®), aluminum hydroxide with magnesium hydroxide (Maalox®, Mylanta®), calcium carbonate (TUMS®, Rolaids®, Titralac®), Alka-Seltzer®, and bismuth subsalicylate (Pepto-Bismol®) are some of the medications available.

Inhibitors for Proton Pumps

The use of proton pump inhibitors (PPIs) is now more common than the use of histamine receptor antagonists. PPIs reduce stomach acid by interfering with an acid-producing enzyme in the stomach wall. GERD, stomach ulcers, and H. pylori are all treated with PPIs (with antibiotics).

Chapter Eleven:
Genitourinary System

Pathophysiology of the Genitourinary System

Incontinence

Urinary incontinence is more frequent in women than in males, and it can range from minor leaks to complete bladder control loss. Involuntary pee leakage caused by sneezing, coughing, laughing, lifting, or exercising is known as stress incontinence. Urge incontinence is the inability to control the urge to urinate regularly. The complete loss of bladder control is referred to as total incontinence.

Hydronephrosis

Hydronephrosis is a sign of a disease in which the kidney pelvis and calyces expand due to a blockage causing urine to be held in the kidney. Symptoms of chronic diseases may not appear until serious kidney damage has occurred. The kidney begins to atrophy with time.

Renal and Ureteral Systems Calculi

Renal and urinary calculi are widespread, especially in men, and can be linked to disorders (hyperparathyroidism, renal tubular acidosis, gout) as well as lifestyle factors including sedentary jobs. Calculi can form at any age, are mostly made of calcium, and range in size from a few microns to more than 6 millimeters. Those with a diameter of less than 4 mm can normally pass through the urine without difficulty.

Acute Tubular Necrosis

Acute tubular necrosis (ATN) occurs when a hypoxic state induces renal ischemia, which destroys the tubular cells of the glomeruli, preventing them from filtering the urine adequately, resulting in acute renal failure.

Acute Kidney Injury

Acute kidney injury (AKI), also known as acute renal failure, is a sudden loss of kidney function that causes decreased renal perfusion, a decrease in glomerular filtration rate, and the accumulation of metabolic waste products (azotemia). Urea, creatinine, and other nitrogen-containing end products accumulate in the bloodstream, resulting in azotemia.

Chronic Kidney Disease

Chronic kidney disease (CKD) develops when the kidneys are unable to filter and eliminate wastes, concentrate urine, or maintain electrolyte balance as a result of hypoxic circumstances, renal disease, or urinary tract obstruction. It causes azotemia (an increase in nitrogenous waste in the blood) before leading to uremia (nitrogenous wastes cause toxic symptoms.)

Uremic Syndrome

End-stage renal disease and renal failure can cause uremic syndrome, which is characterized by several metabolic failures and a drop in creatinine clearance to less than 10 mL/min. Reduced RBC production, platelet abnormalities, metabolic acidosis, hyperkalemia, renal bone disease, numerous endocrine problems, cardiovascular disorders, and anorexia, and malnutrition are all metabolic abnormalities linked to uremia.

Pyelonephritis

Pyelonephritis is a bacterial infection of the kidney parenchyma that can cause organ damage. Pyelonephritis can lead to the creation of abscesses, sepsis, and renal failure.

Cystitis

Cystitis is a common and often-chronic low-grade kidney infection that develops over time, so it's critical to keep an eye out for symptoms of urinary infections and treat them as soon as possible. Urine changes in appearance, color, odor, output, discomfort, and systemic effects.

Nephrotoxic Agents

Medications, particularly in older people, are a significant cause of kidney impairment. If the medicine is stopped before irreversible damage develops, the nephrotoxic effects may be reversed.

Paraphimosis and Phimosis

Both phimosis and paraphimosis are limiting conditions of the penis that affect males who are either uncircumcised or have been circumcised wrongly. The inability to retract the foreskin proximal to the glans penis causes phimosis, which can lead to urine retention or hematuria. When the foreskin thickens above the glans penis and cannot be expanded to its natural position, it is called paraphimosis.

Testicular Torsion

Testicular torsion occurs when the spermatic cord twists within or below the inguinal canal, obstructing blood flow to the testis.

Epididymitis And Orchitis

Epididymitis, or infection of the epididymis, is frequently linked to testicular infection (epididymo-orchitis). Infection in children may be linked to congenital abnormalities that allow urine to reflux. It is generally linked to STDs in sexually active males 35 years or younger. It's typically linked to urinary infections or benign prostatic hypertrophy with urethral blockage in males over 40.

Prostatitis

Prostatitis is an infection of the prostate gland caused by bacteria such as E. coli, Pseudomonas aeruginosa, Staphylococcus aureus, and others. Fever, chills, lower back pain, urine frequency dysuria, painful ejaculation, and perineal soreness are some of the symptoms.

Benign Prostatic Hypertrophy

After the age of 40, benign prostatic hypertrophy/hyperplasia develops. The prostate may gradually increase, but the surrounding tissue prevents outward expansion, causing the urethra to become compressed. The bladder wall changes as well, becoming thicker and inflamed to the point where it spasms, resulting in frequent urination. The bladder muscle weakens over time, and the bladder does not entirely empty.

Pelvic Inflammatory Diseases (PID)

Salpingitis, endometritis, tubo-ovarian abscess, peritonitis, and perihepatitis are examples of diseases of the upper reproductive system that commonly arise from the vaginal and cervix. Most infections are caused by Neisseria gonorrhoeae and Chlamydia trachomatis, but some infections are polymicrobial.

Vulvovaginitis

Inflammation of the vulvar and vaginal tissues is called vulvovaginitis.

Bacterial vaginosis is a type of bacterial vaginosis that affects women (Gardnerella vaginalis or other bacteria).

- Yeast infections (usually Candida albicans)
- Infections with parasites (Trichomonas vaginalis)
- Contact vaginitis due to an allergic reaction (from soaps or other irritants)
- Atrophic vaginitis is a type of atrophic vaginitis (post menopause).

Ovarian Cysts

Ovarian cysts can develop inside or outside the ovaries. A functional cyst develops when a normal monthly follicle continues to grow. There are two types of functional cysts:

- When a follicle does not rupture or release its egg but instead continues to grow, it forms a follicular cyst.
- When fluid builds up inside the follicle after the egg is released, a corpus luteum cyst forms.

Cystadenomas, endometriomas, and dermoid cysts are some of the other forms of ovarian cysts. Multiple cysts can be found in polycystic ovaries.

Bartholin Cysts

The Bartholin glands are tiny glands found in the lips of the labia minora on both sides of the vagina. The glands serve to keep the vulvar area lubricated. When a duct to one gland becomes obstructed, usually due to illness or trauma, a Bartholin cyst develops. resulting in edema and cyst development (usually 1 to 3 cm but may be much larger with infection).

Procedures and Interventions in the Genitourinary System

Renal Dialysis

Peritoneal dialysis. Renal dialysis is reserved for patients who have progressed from renal insufficiency to uremia as a result of end-stage renal disease (ESRD). It could potentially be used only temporarily to treat acute problems. People can be kept alive on dialysis, but because of the numerous difficulties that come with it, many people are considering renal transplantation. Peritoneal dialysis can be done in a variety of ways, including peritoneal dialysis, continuous ambulatory peritoneal dialysis, and continuous cyclic peritoneal dialysis.

Hemodialysis. For patients with ESRD, hemodialysis, the most prevalent type of dialysis, is used for both short-term and long-term dialysis. Hemodialysis is commonly used for patients who are unable to tolerate peritoneal dialysis or who live near a dialysis facility, but it interferes with work or school attendance and necessitates stringent dietary and fluid restrictions in between sessions. Shorter dialysis sessions allow for greater independence, and the higher expenditures may be mitigated by reduced morbidity.

Continuous Renal Replacement Therapy

The blood is circulated by hydrostatic pressure across a semipermeable membrane in continuous renal replacement therapy (CCRT). It is used in critical care and is simple to implement:

- Continuous arteriovenous hemofiltration (CAVH)
- Continuous arteriovenous hemodialysis (CAVHD)
- Continuous venovenous hemofiltration (CVVH)
- Continuous venovenous hemodialysis

Radical Nephrectomy

For adenocarcinoma of the kidney, which may be accompanied by paraneoplastic syndromes and, because this type of cancer is linked to smoking, patients may have underlying coronary artery or pulmonary illness, a radical nephrectomy is performed. Some individuals have erythrocytosis, but many are anemic and may require transfusions to reach a hemoglobin level of >10 g/dL before surgery. If the renal cell carcinoma is less than 4 cm in diameter, nephron-sparing surgery (partial nephrectomy) may be performed, generally using laparoscopy. Analgesia and pulmonary hygiene are needed after surgery.

Bladder Training

Bladder training normally necessitates keeping a toileting diary for at least three days to analyze patterns. There are several techniques to consider:

- Toileting on a set schedule
- Creating a new habit
- Prompted voiding
- Bladder retraining

Bowel Training

Maintaining a stool diary to track progress, as well as scheduled defecation, stimulation, positioning, straining, exercise, and kegel exercises, are all part of bowel training for defecation.

Chapter Twelve:
Musculoskeletal System

Pathophysiology of the Musculoskeletal System

Immobility

Patients in critical care are frequently immobile for long periods, which increases their risk of skin breakdown and the development of pressure ulcers, DVT, functional decline, decreased muscle mass, impaired coordination and gait, cardiovascular deconditioning, depression, and constipation. To avoid the negative impacts of immobility, patients should be reviewed daily for their preparedness to proceed toward their mobility goals.

Gait Disorders

Functional movement disorders are characterized by the involuntary, aberrant movement of a bodily part whose cause is unknown. The most common type of functional movement disorder is functional tremors. Other types of functional movement disorders include dystonia, myoclonus, and Parkinsonism.

Falls

In the hospital context, falls are the most common adverse event. Confusion and agitation are two variables that enhance the chance of falling. Furthermore. Additional risk factors include impaired balance or gait, orthostatic hypotension, reduced mobility, a history of falling, senior age, and the use of certain drugs.

Carpal Tunnel Syndrome

The median nerve is compressed by thickening of the flexor tendon sheath, skeletal encroachment, or a mass in the soft tissue, resulting in carpal tunnel syndrome.

Infectious Arthritis

Bacterial, viral (rubella, parvovirus, and hepatitis B), parasitic, or fungal infections can cause infectious arthritis. The most rapid deterioration of the joint is caused by bacterial arthritis. The most prevalent bacterial agents are Neisseria gonorrhoeae (the most common), Staphylococcus, Streptococcus, and Escherichia coli. The infection could be bloodborne, or it could spread from an infection near the joint, or it could spread via direct implantation or postoperative site contamination. In most cases, the infection affects only one joint.

Tendinitis and Bursitis

Bursitis is a condition in which the bursa becomes inflamed. Bursae are fluid-filled sacs that form in tissues to minimize friction, leading the lining of the bursal walls to thicken. Infection, trauma, crystal deposits, or prolonged friction from trauma can all cause this.

Inflammation of the long, tubular tendons and tendon sheaths close to the bursa is known as tendinitis. Tendonitis has similar causes to bursitis, but it can also be induced by quinolone antibiotics. Both the bursa and the tendons are frequently irritated. Shoulder, olecranon (elbow), trochanteric (hip), and prepatellar bursitis are all common kinds of bursitis (front of the knee). Wrist, Achilles, patellar, and rotator cuff are all common types of tendinitis

Effusion and Arthrocentesis in Conjunction

The collection of fluid (clear, bloody-red, or purulent) within a joint capsule is known as joint effusion. Joint effusion can cause considerable discomfort and pressure on the joint. Arthrocentesis reduces pressure, and the aspirated fluid can be analyzed for diagnostic purposes. In the absence of a referral to an orthopedic expert, arthrocentesis is usually contraindicated in the presence of an underlying infection, a prosthetic joint, or coagulopathy.

Pain in the Lumbosacral System

Strain, muscular weakness, osteoarthritis, spinal stenosis, herniated discs, vertebral fractures, bone metastases, infection, or other musculoskeletal problems can all cause lumbar (low back) pain. The pressure from a disk herniation or other joint abnormalities puts strain on nerves exiting the spinal cord, causing pain to spread along the nerve. Acute or persistent pain might occur (more than 3 months).

Strain and Sprain

A strain occurs when a part of the musculature ("pulled muscle") is overstretched, causing microscopic tears in the muscle. It usually occurs as a result of excessive stress or overuse of the muscle. The onset of discomfort is usually abrupt, with local sensitivity when the muscle is used. A sprain is an injury to a joint that results in a partial rupture of the supporting ligaments, which is commonly caused by twisting or wrenching during a fall.

Injuries to the Joints Caused by High Energy

Low-energy injuries include those sustained from a fall from a standing position or a height of less than one meter, whereas high-energy injuries include those sustained from a larger impact, such as those sustained in an automobile accident, a fall from a greater height, sports accidents (downhill skiing, ice hockey), as well as gunshot wounds, stab wounds, and blast injuries. High-energy injuries are more likely to be serious. and may consist of:

Dislocations and Fractures

Fractures and dislocations are most commonly caused by trauma, such as falls and car accidents, although pathologic fractures can develop when diseased bones, such as those with osteoporosis or metastatic tumors, are subjected to little force. Repetitive trauma, such as forced marching, causes stress fractures. In growing youngsters, salter fractures affect the cartilaginous epiphyseal plate near the ends of long bones. Bone growth can be hampered if this area is damaged. The following are some of the more serious orthopedic injuries:

Pelvic Fracture

Depending on the degree and type of fracture, pelvic fractures can be relatively innocuous or life-threatening. They are most commonly caused by high-speed trauma from car accidents or skiing mishaps.

Osteomyelitis

Osteomyelitis is a bone infection that can result from an open fracture or from an infection that has spread throughout the body. Wounds or soft tissue infections that have developed and spread to the bone can also produce osteomyelitis.

Compartment Syndrome

When the amount of pressure within a grouping of muscles, nerves, and blood arteries increases, the blood flow to the muscles and nerves is disrupted, resulting in compartment syndrome. This is a life-threatening situation. Tissue ischemia and eventual tissue death will result if not treated.

Rhabdomyolysis

When the cells of the skeletal muscles are damaged, toxins from the wounded cells are released into the bloodstream, resulting in rhabdomyolysis.

Interventions and Procedures for Musculoskeletal Disorders

Extremity Compartment Syndrome Monitoring Devices

The 5 P's are symptoms of extremities compartment syndrome:

1. Extreme pain that is out of proportion to the damage
2. Paresthesia
3. Pallor
4. Paresis
5. Pulse deficit

Pressure is usually measured with a device designed for the purpose, although it can also be done with a manometer attached to a needle and syringe.

Pelvic Stabilizer

Pelvic stabilizers are used to stop excessive bleeding from pelvic fractures, keep the bones in the proper position, and avoid additional injury. Bleeding is often reduced by maintaining pressure and minimizing the fracture.

Immobilization Devices

Cervical collars, cervical extrication splints, backboards, full-body splints, various forms of extremity splints, and pneumatic anti-shock garments are examples of immobilization devices (PASG).

Spinal Immobilization

Numbness, tingling, weakness, paralysis, pain or tenderness in the spine, spinal deformity, blunt trauma associated with alterations of consciousness, and high energy injuries associated with drugs/alcohol, the inability of the patient to communicate, and/or distracting injury are now the only indications for spinal immobilization with backboard.

Fractures and Dislocations Immobilization

For fractures and dislocations, immobilization procedures include:

- CAST: After reduction, plaster and fiberglass casts are used to check that the bone is properly aligned
- SPLINT: Plaster splints are made up of 12 or more layers of plaster that have been measured to the exact length and numerous layers of cushioning (longer and wider than splint should be measured and cut).

Care for Amputation

Partially or completely amputations are possible. The severed limb should be handled as if it might be reattached or revascularized at first. Except for the thumb, single digits are frequently not reattached.

Tourniquets

Tourniquets are used to stop bleeding in an extremity and should be used as soon as possible if there is an arterial bleed or if the pressure does not stop the bleeding.

Instruction on how to Walk with Crutches for Patients

Before attempting ambulation, a patient's crutches should be appropriately adjusted. If the patient is only partially or completely weight-bearing, a demonstration should be offered. Stair climbing should be done regularly.

Rehabilitation and Functional Status

ADLs (activities of daily living) are a series of activities used to assess a patient's return to normal function; these are tasks that the patient did every day before hospitalization and will be expected to do once rehabilitation is done.

Rehabilitation

Rehabilitation is a branch of medicine dedicated to assisting patients in regaining and/or restoring functions and abilities following a disease or accident.

Occupational Therapy

Occupational therapy is defined as the application of creative activities to the treatment of people who are disabled, whether physically or intellectually.

Assistive Technology

Before the client begins ambulation, crutches should be correctly adjusted. A cane should be handled in the hand opposite the injured side. The client should be able to propel the walker forward without leaning over to use it.

Chapter Thirteen: **Integument**

Pathophysiology of the Integument

Cellulitis

Cellulitis occurs when an infected region of the skin develops, usually as a result of a skin injury or trauma. Staphylococcus or streptococcus bacteria are the most common causes of cellulitis.

Septic Arthritis

SEPTIC ARTHRITIS is a type of Septic arthritis caused by bacteria, viruses, or fungus invading the joint area.

Extravasation

Extravasation occurs when a vesicant medicine or fluid injected intravenously seeps from the vein into the subcutaneous region. Vesicant drugs are those that, if extravasated, cause tissue harm and, in the worst-case scenario, tissue necrosis.

Tissue Damages Related to the Allergic Contact Dermatitis

Contact dermatitis is a localized allergic reaction that manifests as a rash that may blister and itch. Poison oak, poison ivy, latex, benzocaine, nickel, and preservatives are common allergies, although people can react to a wide range of objects, preparations, and products.

Pressure Ulcers

When the weight of the body exerts pressure on the skin, it reduces perfusion, reducing arterial and capillary blood flow and resulting in ischemia. Ulcers can form as a result of pressure, shearing, and friction.

Infectious Wounds

Infected wounds can occur in a variety of settings. Infectious wounds are a common source of medical attention. Sepsis, multisystem organ failure, and death are all risks associated with wound infections.

Necrotizing Fasciitis

Necrotizing fasciitis is an infection that starts deep inside the fascia and spreads quickly, resulting in tissue necrosis and the death of soft tissue and nerves.

Surgical Wounds

Surgical wounds or incisions are created in a sterile, controlled setting during a surgical procedure.

Tissue Damage

- Abrasion is damage to the skin's surface layers, such as road burn or ligature marks.
- A contusion occurs when friction or pressure causes bruising by damaging the underlying vessels.
- Laceration is a skin tear caused by blunt force, such as falls on protuberances like elbows or other blunt trauma. Lacerations can range from partial to complete thickness.
- An avulsion is a tissue that has been detached from its base and is either missing or does not have a sufficient basis for attachment.

Medical Maggots for Biological Wound Debridement

The open wound is treated with medical maggots, and the peri-wound tissue must be safeguarded. After 48 hours, the maggots are removed from the wound and the area is treated with regular saline.

Pharmacology of the Integumentary System

Anesthetics For Wound Pain on the Skin

Topical anesthetics are one form of pain medicine that can be used to control pain from wounds. During debridement or dressing changes, 2-4 percent lidocaine is commonly utilized. Lidocaine is only good on the surface, and it can take 15-30 minutes for it to take action. The Eutectic Mixture of Local Anesthetics (EMLA Cream) offers effective pain relief. After cleaning the wound, thick layers of cream are applied to the peri-wound tissue.

Wound Pain: Regional Anesthesia

Local anesthetic (injectable subcutaneous and perineural medicines) or nerve blocks are used to treat the wound. Lidocaine, bupivacaine, and tetracaine in solution are among the medications available. To promote vasoconstriction and minimize bleeding, epinephrine is sometimes used. The anesthetic is injected into the peri-wound tissue or wound borders for field blocking. Single injections may be used in regional nerve blocks, which have a short-term impact but can give pain relief throughout therapy.

Chapter Fourteen: **Ear, Nose, and Throat**

Pathophysiology of the Ear, Nose, and Throat

Abscess Peritonsillar

Cellulitis proceeds to abscess between the palatine tonsil and capsule in a peritonsillar abscess (PTA), which is generally caused by tonsillitis. It's frequently polymicrobial. Between the ages of 20 and 30, it frequently occurs bilaterally. Obstruction of the airway, rupture with an aspiration of purulent material, septicemia, endocarditis, and epiglottitis are all possible complications. Polymicrobial infections are common. Fever, discomfort, hoarseness, muffling of the voice, dysphagia, tonsillar edema, erythema, exudate, and edema of the palate with uvula displacement are some of the symptoms.

Recurrent Epistaxis

Recurrent epistaxis is prevalent in young children (2-10 years), particularly males, and is commonly caused by nose-picking, a dry climate, or the use of central heating during the winter. NSAIDs and anticoagulants may be to blame for the rise in incidence between the ages of 50 and 80.

The Kiesselbach plexus in the anterior nares is densely packed with veins and easily bleeds. Bleeding in the posterior nares is more serious and can lead to a significant loss of blood. Blood from the anterior nares normally stays in one nostril, whereas blood from the posterior nares might flow through both nostrils or backward into the throat, causing the person to swallow.

Bell's Palsy

Bell's palsy is a condition that affects only one side of the paired nerves and is caused by inflammation of cranial nerve VII, which is usually caused by a herpes simplex I or II infection. The onset is usually abrupt, and symptoms peak after 48 hours, with a wide spectrum of symptoms. Symptoms normally go away in two to six months, although they might last up to a year.

Temporal Arteritis (TA)

Temporal Arteritis is a condition that affects the arteries in the brain. It is also known as giant cell arteritis and is an inflammation of the blood vessels in the brain, particularly the temporal artery, as well as the aorta and branches of the thoracic aorta. TA is most usually related to polymyalgia rheumatica (30% or less of patients), although it can also occur with other systemic diseases such as lupus erythematosus, Sjogren syndrome, and rheumatoid arthritis. TA is a degenerative condition that can lead to blindness and affects people over the age of 50.

Neuralgia of the Trigeminal System

Trigeminal neuralgia (tic douloureux) is a neurological disorder in which blood vessels press against the trigeminal nerve as it exits the brainstem, causing severe facial or jaw pain. Shock-like aches might affect a small area, half of the face, or both sides of the face at different times. Movement, vibration, or contact with the face or lips can trigger the agony, which lasts anywhere from seconds to two minutes and is quite debilitating.

Ludwig Angina

Ludwig angina is cellulitis of the submandibular spaces and lingual space caused by Streptococcus or Staphylococcus, which can obstruct the airway as the swelling in the mouth floor pushes the tongue superior and posterior.

Externa Otitis

Otitis externa is a bacterial or fungal infection of the external ear canal. Bacteria such as Pseudomonas aeruginosa and Staphylococcus aureus and fungi such as Aspergillus and Candida are common pathogens. Chlorine in swimming pools frequently causes OE by killing regular flora and allowing other germs to grow. Immune problems, diabetes, and steroid use have all been linked to fungal infections.

Medial Otitis

Otitis media, or middle ear inflammation, commonly occurs after upper respiratory tract infections or allergic rhinitis. The eustachian tube swells, preventing air from passing through. Mucous membrane fluid leaks into the middle ear, producing an infection. Streptococcus pneumoniae, Hemophilus influenzae, and Moraxella catarrhalis are all common pathogens. Some genetic diseases, including trisomy 21 and cleft palate, can cause eustachian tube anomalies, raising the risk. Acute, recurrent, bullous, and chronic are the four types.

Mastoiditis

Because the mucous membranes of the middle ear are connected to the mastoid air cells in the temporal bone, mastoiditis is frequently caused by the expansion of acute otitis media. Mastoiditis should be considered in all patients with otitis media. Chronic otitis media patients are more likely to develop chronic mastoiditis, which can lead to the formation of benign cholesteatoma. Mastoiditis is characterized by prolonged fever, pain in or behind the ear (particularly at night), and hearing loss.

Sinusitis

Sinusitis is an inflammation of the nasal sinuses divided into four ethmoidal air cells: two maxillary, two frontal, and one sphenoidal. Inflammation generates drainage obstruction, which produces discomfort.

Disease of Meniere

Meniere's disease is caused by a blockage in the inner ear's endolymphatic duct, which results in dilation of the endolymphatic space and an unbalanced fluid balance, causing pressure or rupture of the inner ear membrane.

Labyrinthitis

Labyrinthitis is an inflammation of the inner ear caused by a virus or bacteria, and it can be caused by bacterial otitis media. Mumps, rubella, rubeola, influenza, and other viral illnesses, such as upper respiratory tract infections, can all cause viral labyrinthitis. Labyrinthitis causes balance problems because the labyrinth contains the vestibular system, which is responsible for sense head movement. The disease usually lasts for 1 to 6 weeks, with acute symptoms in the first week and then diminishing symptoms in the second week.

Temporomandibular Disorder (TMD)

Jaw pain caused by dysfunction of the temporomandibular joint (TMJ) and supporting muscles and ligaments is known as temporomandibular disorder (TMD). It can be triggered by an injury, like whiplash, or by teeth grinding or clenching, stress, or arthritis.

Chapter Fifteen:
Multiple Systems

Pathophysiology of Multiple Systems

Severe Infection Range

Severe infections are referred to by a variety of names, many of which are interchangeable. These terms must be understood to complete the continuum of care correctly.

- Bacteremia is defined as the presence of bacteria in the bloodstream without the presence of a systemic infection.
- Septicemia is a systemic infection caused by organisms in the blood (typically bacteria or fungus).
- The systemic inflammatory response syndrome (SIRS) is a systemic inflammatory reaction that affects multiple organ systems. Elevated tachypnea, tachycardia, and leukocytosis are all symptoms of SIRS.
- Sepsis is an infection with a broad life-threatening inflammatory response that can occur locally or systemically (SIRS).
- Indications of SIRS and sepsis, as well as signs of growing organ dysfunction with inadequate perfusion and/or hypotension, are all signs of severe sepsis.

- Septic shock is a condition that develops after severe sepsis and is marked by resistant hypotension despite therapy. Lactic acidosis symptoms may be present.
- The most common cause of sepsis-related death is multi-organ dysfunction syndrome (MODS). Acute respiratory distress syndrome (ARDS) can develop, and renal failure can occur as a result of acute tubular necrosis or cortical necrosis. About 30% of those who are affected develop thrombocytopenia, which can lead to disseminated intravascular coagulation (DIC). You may get liver damage and intestinal necrosis.

Shock

There are many distinct types of shocks. However, there are several qualities that they all share. Hypotension causes a significant decrease in tissue perfusion, resulting in insufficient oxygen delivery to the tissues and inadequate removal of cellular waste products, resulting in tissue injury: hypotension, decreased urinary output, metabolic acidosis, peripheral/cutaneous vasoconstriction/vasodilation, and changes in the level of consciousness are all symptoms of shock.

The following are the different types of shock:

- **Distributive:** Preload is decreased, CO is increased, SVR is decreased
- **Cardiogenic:** Preload is increased, CO is decreased, SVR is increased
- **Hypovolemic:** Preload is decreased, CO is decreased, SVR is increased

N/B: (CO) is cardiac output, (SVR) is systemic vascular resistance

Distributive Shock

Because of arterial/venous dilatation, which results in lower vascular tone and hypoperfusion of internal organs, distributive shock occurs when blood volume is adequate but intravascular volume is insufficient. Cardiac output could be normal or blood could pool and reduce cardiac output. Anaphylactic shock, septic shock, neurogenic stress, and medication ingestions can all cause distributed shock.

Neurogenic Shock

Neurogenic shock is a kind of distributive shock that happens when the autonomic nervous system, which governs the cardiovascular system, is damaged by trauma resulting in acute spinal cord injury (including blunt and piercing injuries), neurological illnesses, medications, or anesthesia.

Anaphylactic Shock

Anaphylactic shock or anaphylactic reaction might have only a few symptoms or a vast variety of potentially fatal consequences. After the initial therapy (biphasic anaphylaxis), symptoms may reappear, thus close monitoring is required.

Volume Deficit/Hypovolemic Shock

When there is insufficient intravascular fluid, hypovolemic shock ensues. Massive hemorrhage, heat injuries, severe vomiting or diarrhea, and internal injuries (such as ruptured spleen or dissecting arteries) that interfere with intravascular integrity can all result in total fluid loss. Hypovolemia can also be caused by vasodilation, increased capillary membrane permeability as a result of sepsis or trauma, and lower colloidal osmotic pressure (which can occur with sodium loss and certain spleen or dissecting arteries) that compromise intravascular integrity.

Syndrome of Post-Intensive Care

PICS refers to the disabilities that occur as a result of intensive care therapy for severe diseases, such as coronavirus patients who have been in an induced coma for weeks and have been on mechanical breathing. The following are some of the impairments:

- **Cognitive:** Difficulty speaking, memory loss, concentration problems, and executive dysfunction
- **Psychological:** Depression, anxiety, PTSD, delirium, and a lack of motivation are all psychological issues. PICS can also affect family members and caregivers as a result of the emotional stress they face, which is most commonly seen with psychological issues (grief, anxiety, depression, insomnia, PTSD)
- **Physical** symptoms include generalized weakness, dyspnea, sleeplessness, lethargy, weariness, and walking difficulties.

Hyperthermia Malignant

Malignant hyperthermia is a potentially fatal illness caused by a hereditary predisposition to inhalational anesthetics (except nitrous oxide and succinylcholine). Large, strong muscles, as well as a history of unexplained fevers or a family history of death after surgery, are all risk factors.

Hypothermia

Hypothermia occurs when the core body temperature falls below 95 °F (35 °C) as a result of exposure to cold conditions. Hypothermia can be caused by immersion in cold water, exposure to cold temperatures, metabolic diseases (hypothyroidism, hypoglycemia, hypoadrenalism), or abnormalities in the central nervous system (CNS) (head trauma, Wernicke disease). Many hypothermia patients are under the influence of alcohol or narcotics.

- Pallor, cold skin, drowsiness, and changes in mental status are all signs of hypothermia.
- There was a lot of confusion and a lot of shivering. Shock, unconsciousness, and dysrhythmias (T-waves) are all possible outcomes.
- PR, QRS, and QT inversion and prolongation), as well as atrial fibrillation and AV block, and cardiac arrest.

Multisystem Interventions and Procedures

Temperature Monitoring Continuously

Temperature monitoring can be done in a variety of ways, including:

- Catheter for the pulmonary artery (most accurate but generally not recommended because of invasiveness and potential for complications)
- Temperature probes, either rectal or Foley
- Probes for the skin
- Bluetooth monitors that are worn on the skin and transfer data to an external monitor or the patient's electronic health record.

Permissive Hypotension

Permissive hypotension procedures allow the systolic blood pressure to drop low enough to prevent or control hemorrhage while keeping the perfusion high enough. While it comes to trauma patients, this entails limiting fluid resuscitation when there is active bleeding. Permissive hypotension is defined as a systolic blood pressure of less than 80 mmHg, though this can change depending on the procedure.

Sedation

Minimal sedation. Local/topical anesthesia, peripheral nerve blocks, injection of 50 percent nitrogen oxide in oxygen alone, or administration of one sedative or analgesic medicine in a dosage that does not generally require supervision are all examples of minimal sedation. The goal of minimum sedation is to diminish pain perception, relax the patient, and alleviate anxiety. Throughout the procedure, the patient's level of consciousness, sedation, and discomfort should be checked to ensure that the dosage is appropriate and that the patient is not overly sedated.

Continuous vs. Intermittent. For severely ill individuals, sedation may include:

- **Intermittent sedation** is a type of sedation that is delivered via IV push and has a short duration. Benzodiazepines and opioids are common agents. Intermittent sedation is most commonly used for endoscopic operations, but it is also occasionally used for patients on artificial ventilators, particularly if they are undergoing regular weaning trials.
- **Continuous sedation** is sedation that is delivered via a continuous intravenous infusion and lasts longer. Opioids, midazolam, and propofol are common agents. Because it requires less intervention and maintains a constant blood level, continuous sedation is more routinely utilized for patients on mechanical ventilation. As an experiment for weaning patients off mechanical ventilation, daily breaks of continuous sedation could be used.

Neuromuscular Blockade Agents: Neuromuscular blockers are used to produce paralysis in patients who have not reacted well to sedation, particularly for intubation and mechanical ventilation. Because NMBAs do not cause unconsciousness, amnesia, or analgesia, they must be given only after the patient has been thoroughly sedated. Depolarizing and non-depolarizing agents are both NMBAs.

Sedation With Consciousness. The ASA sedation guidelines (2018) are intended for procedures requiring moderate (conscious) sedation, such as colonoscopy. The following are the steps to take:

Propofol-Based sedation. Propofol is frequently used in sedation for a drug-induced coma. Propofol is the most commonly used non-opioid hypnotic anesthetic for induction. It's also utilized for postoperative sedation and maintenance.

Emergence Delayed

Delayed emergence (failure to emerge for 30-60 minutes after anesthetic agents have worn off) is more common in the elderly due to slowed anesthetic agent metabolism, but it can occur for a variety of reasons, including drug overdose during surgery, pre-induction drug overdose, or alcohol that potentiates intraoperative drugs.

Complications of the Respiratory System After Anesthesia

Because postoperative respiratory problems are most likely during the postanesthesia period, it's crucial to keep an eye on oxygen levels to avoid hypoxemia:

- Partial or complete obstruction of the airway is possible.
- Hypoventilation (PaCO >45 mmHg) is usually minor, although it can result in respiratory acidosis.
- Hypoxemia (mild) is generally associated with hypoventilation and/or enhanced right-to-left shunting.

Cardiovascular Complications After Anesthesia

After surgery, cardiovascular issues are frequently linked to pulmonary complications, which may require treatment as well. The following are some of the complications:

- Most cases of hypotension are minor and do not require treatment.
- Those with a history of hypertension are more likely to develop hypertension 30 minutes following surgery.
- Arrhythmias are mainly caused by respiratory problems or the effects of anesthetics.

Viral Infections

Herpes Simplex Virus Infections

Human herpesvirus 1 and 2 are two kinds of herpes simplex virus (HSV). HSV-1 is usually transmitted through intimate contact and causes gingivostomatitis (also known as "cold sores" or "fever blisters"). The sexual encounter with HSV-2 frequently results in painful genital lesions. Both of these substances can be found in different parts of the body.

Epstein-Barr Infection

The Epstein-Barr virus (EBV) is a type of herpes virus (human herpesvirus 4) that causes infectious mononucleosis. It remains dormant in B cells and epithelial cells after the initial infection. Certain epithelial and lymphatic neoplasms have been linked to it (e.g., nasopharyngeal carcinoma, Burkitt lymphoma, Hodgkin lymphoma).

Mumps, Measles, and Rubella

The **rubeola** (measles) virus is highly contagious, spreads by respiratory secretions (incubation is 7-14 days), and is most common in late winter and early spring. It starts with a high fever (4-7 days), cough, congestion, and conjunctivitis, followed by Koplik spots (pathognomonic), and subsequently a maculopapular rash (spreads cephalocaudally). Notify the health department right away if you detect a case. A positive IgM antibody test (taken after 3 days of rash), viral culture, or PCR can be used to confirm the diagnosis. Treatment is reassuring.

Mumps (parotitis) is a viral infection communicated through saliva (incubation period: 12-24 days). It is most common in the winter and spring. It causes painful salivary gland enlargement (parotid). Report to the health department. Supportive treatment. Orchitis (infertility), pancreatitis, and meningitis are all complications.

Rubella (German measles) is a virus that spreads through respiratory droplets and peaks in the spring (incubation time: 2-3 weeks). There is a slight prodrome (fever, pains, sore throat, conjunctivitis, swollen nodes [esp. suboccipital, postauricular, & posterior cervical]), then a maculopapular rash (face 15 then down) (face 15 then down). Report to the health department. IgM or IgG rubella antibodies should be used to confirm the diagnosis. Symptomatic treatment.

Influenza

Influenza is a highly contagious virus that attacks the respiratory system from the nose to the lungs. The influenza virus is divided into three types: A (which causes epidemics), B (which exclusively affects humans), and C. Types A and B are the most prevalent and are the viruses against which the yearly flu vaccine is most effective; type C is less common and less severe.

Coronavirus

A coronavirus is a common virus that produces cough, runny nose, sore throat, and congestion, among other symptoms. The majority of coronavirus instances aren't harmful, and they go undiscovered most of the time. However, two world-wide pandemics have been caused by distinct coronavirus strains. SARS (severe acute respiratory syndrome) was the first to manifest in China in 2002 and soon spread over the world. It was highly contagious, easily transmitting from person to person through close contact by contaminated droplets produced by coughing or sneezing. SARS was also extremely dangerous, with a case mortality rate of over 10%. Infection rates were high among healthcare personnel and anyone who came into touch with infected patients, necessitating quick identification and isolation. By 2004, there had been no active cases of SARS documented.

The COVID-19 strain, which initially surfaced in December 2019 in the Chinese city of Wuhan and quickly spread around the world, was the most recent coronavirus outbreak. COVID-19 has a similar presentation to SARS, with the remarkable addition of abrupt loss of taste/smell as a distinct identifier. There's still a lot we don't know about this breed, including its specific origins.

Methods of transmission (albeit droplet transmission is hypothesized), effective treatment protocols, and long-term impacts are also factors to consider.

Cytomegalovirus

Cytomegalovirus (CMV) is a herpes virus that affects nearly everyone by the time they reach adulthood. Transmission can occur through secretions from the mother to the newborn before, during, or after birth, as well as through physical contact. The majority of instances are asymptomatic, but a few infants may experience prenatal harm such as jaundice, hepatitis, brain impairment, or growth retardation.

Syncytial Respiratory Virus

The respiratory syncytial virus (RSV) attacks the respiratory system and causes nasal congestion, cough, sore throat, and headache. Harsh cases might result in a high fever, difficulty breathing, a severe cough, and cyanosis.

Bacteria Infections

Diphtheria. Diphtheria, which is caused by the bacteria Corynebacterium diphtheriae, is most common in the fall and winter. Transmission occurs by direct contact with nasal, ocular, and oral secretions over 2-7 days, possibly longer. Slight fever, nasal discharge, sore throat, feeling sick, poor appetite, and airway edema are all symptoms.

Tetanus. Tetanus is a disease caused by Clostridium tetani that can be found all over the world. The bacillus' spores can be found in dirt, dust, and the gastrointestinal tracts of both animals and humans. The incubation period is three to twenty-one days. Headaches, irritation, jaw muscle spasms, and inability to open the mouth are the first signs. Seizures, incontinence, and fever follow, as do acute back muscle spasms.

Fungal Infections

Cryptococcosis. Cryptococcosis is an infection caused by inhaling the fungus Cryptococcus neoformans, which can be found in soil all over the world (and is linked to bird droppings), or Cryptococcus gattii, which is linked to particular trees in the Northwest.

Histoplasmosis

Inhalation of spores from the fungus Histoplasma capsulatum, which can be found in soil and is associated with bird and bat droppings, causes histoplasmosis (e.g, chicken coops, caves).

Pneumocystis

Pneumocystis jiroveci (formerly Pneumocystis carinii) is a fungus that causes pneumonia (PJP, previously PCP) in immunocompromised people. By the age of three or four, the majority of people had been exposed to it.

Candidal Infection

Candida is a yeast that can cause a range of infections, including:

- Oral thrush is a common occurrence among diabetics and immunocompromised people. Burning on the tongue or in the mouth is common, as are "curd-like" white spots that can be scraped away to reveal crimson tissue underlying. KOH preparation is used to make the diagnosis.
- Candida esophagitis can affect immunocompromised people, and symptoms include dysphasia, odynophagia, and chest pain.
- Candidal intertrigo, often known as diaper rash, causes beefy-red lesions in the skin folds and satellite lesions. Topical antifungals are used to treat the infection.
- Fungal blood cultures are used to identify candidemia, which can cause osteomyelitis, endocarditis, and other problems.

Ringworm

Ringworm is caused by an infection with the Tinea fungus, which results in skin patches with normal cores that resemble a ring.

Infections Caused by Parasitic Vectors

Malaria

Malaria is a blood-borne disease caused by the Plasmodium parasite, which is widespread in tropical locations. There are + bacteria that are known to cause disease in humans (P. malariae, P. vivax, P. ovale, and P. falciparum). The female Anopheles mosquito transmits these protozoa. They replicate in the liver before being discharged and infecting RBCs, where they continue to multiply. Depending on the parasite species, the incubation period might be as little as 9 days or as long as many years.

Lyme Disease

A bite from a deer tick (black-legged tick) infected with the spirochete bacterium Borrelia burgdorferi causes Lyme disease. It is the most common tick-borne disease in the U.S. and is more prevalent in heavily wooded areas. The tick remains attached once it bites; however, the spirochete is transmitted to the person after 36-48 hours for nymphs and 48-72 hours for adults. The incubation period ranges from 3 to 30 days.

Rocky Mountain Spotted Fever

Rickettsia rickettsii causes Rocky Mountain spotted fever, a tick-borne sickness. It usually happens in the spring and summer across the United States. The incubation period lasts around one week. Headache, fever, nausea, vomiting, loss of appetite, muscle soreness, and a rash on the ankles and wrists are some of the symptoms.

Helminth Infestations

Roundworms [nematodes: Ascaris, hookworms (cause anemia), filariae (cause elephantiasis)] and flatworms [tapeworms (cause weight loss); flukes (intestinal or liver)] are among the helminth infestations (woriis). The most prevalent helminth infestation is pinworms, a kind of roundworm that causes enterobiasis. Patients may be asymptomatic or suffer from severe anal itching, which is often greater at night and can lead to insomnia. Abdominal discomfort, nausea, and vomiting are all possible side effects.

Giardia Lamblia

The protozoan Giardia lamblia affects water supplies and spreads to children via the fecal-oral pathway. It is the most prevalent cause of nonbacterial diarrhea in the United States, with around 20,000 cases of infection in people of all ages each year.

Toxoplasmosis

Toxoplasmosis is a parasitic infection caused by Toxoplasma gondii, a parasite typically found in soil. It is ubiquitous and spreads by cat feces; however, it can also be contracted by eating undercooked meat or vegetables that have not been properly washed. Toxoplasmosis is a dangerous infection that can affect a variety of organs. Immunocompromised and pregnant women, as well as their unborn children, are more vulnerable to the disease's side effects (the "T" in congenital TORCH infections).

Fibromyalgia and Fever

Febrile Seizure

A febrile seizure is a type of generalized seizure that occurs between the ages of six months and five years old and is associated with a high fever (usually more than 38°C [100.4°F]) caused by any type of infection (upper respiratory tract, urinary) but without an intracranial infection or other cause. To rule out more serious illnesses, a thorough clinical evaluation is required. Unless an intracranial infection is suspected, lumbar puncture is usually not recommended. Seizures normally last less than 15 minutes and have no lasting effects on the brain.

Fibromyalgia

Fibromyalgia is a multi-symptom illness characterized by fatigue, chronic widespread muscle pain, and specific areas of tenderness that last at least three months. Fibromyalgia has only lately been recognized as a unique condition, and the cause is unknown.

Pain Management Using Pharmacology

WHO Pain Ladder?

The WHO pain ladder is an algorithm for treating pain using drugs that have increasingly higher potencies. Both adult and pediatric patients can benefit from this technique. Starting with the least potent drug, each step increases the strength of the analgesic until the pain is completely relieved.

There are three steps in the WHO pain ladder.

- Step 1: A non-opioid medicine is given to the patient, which can be used alone or in combination with other adjuvant therapy.
- Step 2: If the patient's pain level remains unchanged, mild- to moderate-level pain-relieving opioids are given, along with adjuvants if they have not been given earlier.
- Step 3: For moderate to severe pain, opioids are used to relieve uncontrolled pain. Adjuvants can also be used indefinitely.

Pain Medication Scheduling

Patients with mild to moderate pain can take acetaminophen with an NSAID like ibuprofen regularly or as needed (PRN) at the onset of pain or when pain is expected (such as before a dressing change). Long-acting opioid pain drugs, such as time-released MS Contin, Duragesic, and OxyContin, should be taken regularly around the clock for severe chronic pain because they help not only control but also prevent pain. When the patient is pain-free, he or she should not skip a dose because this makes control more difficult when the pain returns. In addition to regularly scheduled drugs, the patient may require PRN use of short-acting supplemental medications such as Percocet. Instead of waiting until the pain is severe, patients should take short-acting drugs before the commencement of pain, before anticipated pain, or at the onset of increased discomfort. The goal should always be to keep the pain under control.

Treating Breakthrough Pain

The following are the three basic forms of breakthrough pain and their treatment options:

- **Incident Pain:** Pain that can be linked to a single activity or event, such as a clothing change or physical therapy, is known as incident pain. These things can be predicted. Before the unpleasant occurrence, a rapid-onset, short-acting painkiller was administered.
- **Spontaneous Pain:** This form of pain is unpredictably painful and cannot be linked to a certain moment or incident. There's no way to predict when the pain will strike. Adjuvant treatment may be beneficial in the presence of neuropathic pain. Otherwise, short-acting, rapid-onset analgesia is utilized.
- **End-of-Dose Failure:** Pain that occurs at the end of a regular analgesic dosage cycle, when medicine blood levels start to fall. End-of-dose failure can be detected early on and prevented. It could be a sign of increased dose tolerance and the need to adjust drug dosages.

Management of Neuropathic Pain

The procedures used to treat neuropathic pain are frequently different from those used to treat other types of pain. Anticonvulsants, anesthetics, and antidepressants are the three medication types most widely used and proven helpful for treating neuropathic pain. Amitriptyline, nortriptyline, duloxetine, gabapentin, topical lidocaine, opioids, and pregabalin are some of the most commonly prescribed drugs.

Management of Bone Pain

The causal factor for bone pain, such as the original cancer site, severely damaged bones, or fractures, may affect treatment options. Chemotherapy, radiation, and hormone therapy are all options for systemic treatment. When estrogen and androgen receptors are present in cancer cells, hormone treatment is used. Bisphosphonates like ibandronate, zoledronate, and alendronate can strengthen bones, halt deterioration, and prevent fractures while also reducing pain. Fatigue, fever, nausea, vomiting, and anemia are all possible adverse effects. Surgery may be used to remove malignant cells or strengthen fragile bone regions. The most common pain relievers are opioids and NSAIDs/COX-2 inhibitors, which must be given regularly.

Chapter Sixteen: **Geriatric**

Geriatric Pathophysiology

Syndromes of the Geriatric System

Geriatric syndromes are a group of disorders that include the most prevalent non-disease conditions encountered in the geriatric population. Falls, frailty, incontinence, delirium, functional decline, antibodies and immunity, allergies, driving, and rapid eye movement are all essential areas in which the nurse must be knowledgeable (REM)

Incontinence of the Urinary Tract

The involuntary loss of urine is known as urinary incontinence (UI). The rate of occurrence rises with age and is more common in women. Urinary incontinence can be classified as transitory, urge or reflex, stress (SUI), or enuresis.

Changes in the Respiratory System as a Person Ages

The respiratory system of an elderly patient alters in the following ways:

1. The rigidity of the rib cage increases

2. The ability of the chest wall to operate is reduced
3. The size of the trachea and bronchi expands
4. The parenchyma of the lungs is less elastic
5. Coughs aren't as strong and breaths aren't as deep

Common Comorbidities Discussed Among the Elderly

Geriatric comorbidities are a group of chronic or acute disorders that have been linked to a higher death rate in the elderly population, as well as a faster rate of disability aggravation and functional decline. The following are the three most typical comorbidity patterns among the elderly:

- **Heart disease:** MI, coronary artery disease, and congestive heart failure are frequently associated with metabolic disorders such as hypertension, diabetes, obesity, and gout.
- **Anxiety/Depression/Somatoform Disorders and Pain:** Pain (systemic, localized, or joint-related) is frequently associated with psychological problems such as anxiety, depression, and cognitive deterioration. Gastrointestinal problems appear to be linked to several mental illnesses.
- **Neuropsychiatric disorders:** Psychiatric disorders like Parkinson's and dementia are frequently linked to neurological problems like incontinence, vascular problems, and/or nerve pain.

Common Psychological Responses to Chronic Illness

Chronic illnesses present themselves in a variety of ways. Over time, this psychological stress may drive the patient to regress and acquire more infantile responses to chronic sickness. Fear, low self-esteem, and a sense of loss of control are common psychological responses to chronic illnesses.

Pharmacology for the Elderly

Elderly Patient Medication Considerations

Most senior people have at least one chronic health issue, such as arthritis, high blood pressure, heart difficulties, diabetes, or other ailments that require multiple medications to address. Elderly people experience greater adverse drug reactions (ADR), with 10% of them requiring hospitalization to alleviate the side effects. Edema, nausea, vomiting, anorexia, vertigo, loose stools, infrequent and difficult stools, confusion, and urine retention are all common side effects. Make sure you don't mistake these for another aging condition or symptom.

Older Adults' Pharmacokinetics

Absorption, distribution, metabolism, and elimination are the four processes in pharmacokinetics. Because the organs involved degrade with age, all of these steps are affected by the patient's age:

1. The majority of drugs are absorbed in the small intestine. Due to decreasing blood flow to the small intestine, drug absorption in elderly persons may be delayed or reduced. This could affect the medicine levels in the geriatric patient's blood.
2. A change in body composition affects the drug's distribution. Total body water and lean muscle mass are lower in elderly patients. The duration of action of lipid-soluble medicines may be lengthened as a result of this relative increase in total body fat.
3. The liver or the kidneys metabolize the majority of drugs. Decreased function of these organs causes medication metabolism and excretion to be delayed.
4. As people get older, their kidney function and elimination effectiveness deteriorate, making it more difficult for them to remove toxins and medications from the body. As a result, medications may stay in the body longer in the elderly, necessitating fewer doses.

Criteria for Beer

The Beers Criteria, often known as the Beers List, is a set of guidelines for identifying improper pharmaceutical use in older people. The list is used to identify which medications are beneficial to older persons against those that pose a risk.

Difficulties in Medication use may be Experienced by the Elderly Population.

The following are some of the most common medication-related issues among the elderly:

- Prescription drug abuse is rampant.
- Issues with medication adherence and compliance
- Due to challenges with comprehension, hearing, or suitable schooling style, there is a misunderstanding of how the medicine is supposed to be taken.
- Not being able to recall the reason, dosage, or frequency with which the medicines should be taken (may result in repeating the medicine when it has already been taken).
- Having a hard time affording the medication.
- Due to vision problems, you may misunderstand the label and take the incorrect dosage.
- Having trouble opening the bottle, coping with little tablets, halving pills, and utilizing inhalers.
- Using the generic and brand names of the same product at the same time can lead to unintended redundancy of the same drug, similar to how using more than one medical worker or
- More than one pharmacy can lead to inadvertent redundancy of the same medication.

Adverse Reactions to Commonly Used Prescription Medications

Certain physical and psychological conditions may occur as a result of taking prescription medication:

- **Bewilderment:** Digoxin, cimetidine, dopamine agent, antihistamine, hypnotic, sedative, anticholinergic, anticonvulsant
- **Anorexia:** Digoxin
- **Low energy or weakness:** Diuretic, antidepressant, antihypertensive
- **Absentmindedness:** Barbiturate
- **Difficult bowel movements:** Anticholinergic
- **Loose stool:** Oral antacid
- **GI upset:** Iron, NSAID, salicylate, corticosteroid, estrogen, alcohol
- **Ringing in the ears (tinnitus):** Analgesic
- **Urinary retention:** Anticholinergic, alpha-agonist
- **Orthostatic low blood pressure:** Antihypertensive, sedative, diuretic, antidepressant
- **Depression:** Benzodiazepine
- **Vertigo:** Sedative, antihypertensive, anticonvulsant, diuretic

Histamine Blockers, Ibuprofen, and Beta-Blockers: Side Effects

In the elderly, histamine blockers might elicit paradoxical central nervous system stimulation, which can result in ataxia. Antihistamines can cause visual and movement issues, which can lead to falls and unexpected hospital visits, or the need for a nursing home. Antihistamines can potentially reduce the effectiveness of other medications or increase the bad side effects of other medications.

Renal dysfunction is already a problem for certain elderly people. Ibuprofen can exacerbate these conditions, resulting in nephrosis, cirrhosis, and congestive heart failure.

Because the aged patient's beta-adrenergic receptor sensitivity is reduced, a beta-blocker is not a good alternative for treating hypertension in them. Calcium entry antagonists, ACE inhibitors, and diuretics are used in lesser doses in elderly people. A high dose can lead to irritability, impotence, fatigue, and a decreased capacity to think effectively in the elderly.

Polypharmacy

Polypharmacy is a term that refers to the usage of numerous drugs at the same time. It occurs when patients take medications that are not prescribed, medications that have negative interactions with one another, and people take medications that are contraindicated.

Obtain a complete pharmacological history at each appointment to manage polypharmacy and avoid problems. Nonprescription drugs and natural therapies should be included. It is critical to educate patients about the problem of polypharmacy.

Master Guidelines for Rational Drug Therapy

Drugs are often quite helpful and effective in treating ailments, but there comes a point where they become detrimental to the patient. The MASTER guidelines must be remembered by the practitioner while deciding whether or not to utilize a drug.

- **M** stands for reducing the number of drugs a patient is taking to a minimum.
- **A** stands for alternative treatments that may be as effective as or more effective than taking a medicine.
- **S** stands for "start small and gradually increase." Give the patient the bare minimum and proceed with caution when increasing doses.
- **T** stands for titration, which is tailoring the amount of medication given to each patient over time.
- **E** stands for patient education regarding the medications he or she is taking.
- **R** stands for regular drug and dose reviews.

Chapter Seventeen:
Psychosocial

Psychosocial Pathophysiology

Delays in Development and Intellectual Disability

When a patient's mental development lags behind that of the general population, it's called developmental delay. Individuals with intellectual disabilities may struggle to adjust to changing surroundings, require support in decision-making, and have self-care or communication impairments. From shy and passive to hyperactive and violent, there is a wide spectrum of behaviors. Inherited (Tay-Sachs), toxin-related (maternal alcohol intake), perinatal (hypoxia), environmental (lack of stimulation/neglect), or acquired intellectual disability (encephalitis, brain injury). The findings of standardized testing are combined with behavior analysis to make a diagnosis.

The following are the IQ-based classifications for intellectual disabilities:

- **Educable to roughly 6% grade level for those aged 55 to 69 (moderate in 85 percent of cases).** It might not be diagnosed until adolescence. Usually able to pick up new skills and maintain themselves, but may require aid and supervision.

- **40-54 (moderate, 10% of cases).** Trainable and may be able to work and live in supervised or sheltered surroundings.
- **25-39 (severe, 4% of cases).** Language is typically delayed, and students can only master basic academic abilities and complete rudimentary chores.
- **25 (severe, 1-2 percent of cases).** Usually associated with sensorimotor impairment in neurological disorders. Constant attention and supervision are required.

Nursing considerations: Always treat patients based on their developmental level rather than their chronological age. This is especially true when it comes to consent and education. People with developmental delays are more likely to be injured or abused.

Personality Disorder

A personality disorder is a long-term set pattern or trait of conduct that differs from what is expected in a culture. These diseases make it difficult for people to form meaningful interpersonal relationships, feel fulfilled, or enjoy life. The onset of the disease is usually in teens or early adulthood. This attitude is manifested in the form of ideas, feelings, and actions. As a person grows older, his or her behaviors are likely to become less intense.

Groupings Of DSM Classification

The DSM-5 categorizes ten personality disorders into three groups: A, B, and C.

- Disorders in Cluster A are marked by unusual or eccentric behaviors, as well as a proclivity for social awkwardness and seclusion.
- Disorders that are marked by erratic, highly emotional, dramatic, or impulsive behaviors are classified as Cluster B.
- Cluster C illnesses are characterized by a high prevalence of scared or anxious feelings.

Bipolar Disorder

Bipolar disorder is characterized by extreme mood swings between hyperactivity and depression, as well as impaired judgment due to skewed ideas. Because bipolar disease is linked to a high likelihood of suicide, it's crucial to get diagnosed and treated as soon as possible. Both drugs (typically taken regularly) and psychosocial therapy, such as cognitive therapy, are used to help manage aberrant thought patterns and behavior. A psychiatric referral is required.

Depression

Depression is a mood illness that is marked by deep sadness and withdrawal. For at least two weeks, a major depressive episode is defined as a gloomy mood, a profound and consistent sense of hopelessness and despair, or a lack of interest in all or almost all activities. Tricyclic antidepressants (TCAs) and selective serotonin reuptake inhibitors (SSRIs) are both used to treat depression, but SSRIs have fewer negative effects and are less likely to cause mortality in the event of an overdose. Counseling, cognitive behavioral therapy, treatment of the underlying reason, and the implementation of an exercise routine may all assist to alleviate depression.

Anxiety Disorders

Anxiety is a natural human feeling and experience that affects everyone at some point in their lives. During an anxiety reaction, you may experience feelings of doubt, powerlessness, isolation, alienation, and insecurity. Anxiety frequently emerges in the absence of a known object or source. Fatigue, inability to concentrate, impatience, insomnia, restlessness, loss of mental processes or turning blank, and muscle tension are all symptoms that the person will feel.

Peplau identified four distinct levels of anxiousness:

1. The anxiety of a mild kind
2. Moderate anxiety
3. Severe anxiety
4. Panic

Panic Attacks

Panic attacks are short bursts of high anxiety (usually lasting 5-10 minutes) that can cause a variety of symptoms such as dyspnea, palpitations, hyperventilation, nausea and vomiting, great fear or worry, chest discomfort and pressure, vertigo and fainting, and tremors.

A detailed history is necessary since panic attacks can be linked to agoraphobia, depression, or intimate partner violence and abuse (IPVA). Patients typically fear they are dying or suffering a heart attack and require comfort and therapy in the ED for acute episorie, such as diazepam or lorazepam.

PTSD

Patients who have been through a traumatic event may relive the event through uncomfortable thoughts and recollections. Nightmares, flashbacks, sleepless-ness, hyperarousal symptoms such as anger and anxiety, avoidance, and negative thoughts and sentiments about oneself and others are all common symptoms. To assist regulate the symptoms of PTSD, pharmacologic therapy may be used. Group and individual/family therapy, cognitive behavioral therapy, and anxiety management/relaxation strategies are all non-pharmacologic treatment options. Hypnosis is another option.

Stress

The body undergoes a multitude of physical and psychological changes as a result of stress. Lack of oxygen, the presence of poisons or chemicals, and infection are the most prevalent stresses for cells. The cells will become harmed and perish if the stress that caused them to alter persists. Organ and systemic failure occur when enough cells die.

Interventions and Psychosocial Procedures

Modification of Behavior

Behavior modification is a sort of systematic therapy that aims to replace maladaptive behaviors with more beneficial ones. Individuals, organizations, or entire communities can benefit from this sort of therapy. The goal of this strategy is to eliminate undesirable behaviors by using positive reinforcement targeted at desired behaviors.

Therapy for Cognitive-Behavioral Problems

CBT focuses on unlearning old behaviors and learning new ones, as well as questioning actions and doing homework. This type of counseling is usually done for a short time, 12-20 sessions. The early sessions gather information about the client's background, the middle sessions concentrate on the issues, and the final sessions review and reinforce newly acquired habits and cognitive patterns. During the sessions, individuals are given homework to explore new ways of thinking and create new coping techniques.

Model of Recovery

Instead of the physician deciding on a treatment plan, the Recovery Model approach to mental health places control of treatment alternatives in the hands of the patient. The purpose of this paradigm is to provide the patient with more independence so that they can reach their ultimate goals of finding work, housing, and living independently.

Therapy of Acceptance and Commitment

When patients are experiencing anxiety or depression, they are encouraged to evaluate their thought processes (cognitive delusion). Patients are encouraged to analyze their values and manage those things that are under their control, such as their facial expressions or actions, as part of ACT's basic notion of mindfulness. Accepting reactions, choosing a path, and taking action to impact change are all part of the ACT acronym.

Therapy in a Single Session

Single-session therapy is the most common type of counseling since people generally only attend one session for a variety of reasons, even if more are recommended. In one session, the purpose is to identify a problem and come up with a solution. The therapist acts as a catalyst, encouraging the individual to see the problem as part of a larger pattern that can be altered and a solution to be found.

Solution-Focused Therapy

Solution-focused therapy is based on the idea that change is possible, but that the individual must first identify and address problems in the actual world. Questioning is used in this treatment to assist the individual in establishing goals and finding solutions to difficulties.

Nonviolent Crisis Intervention and De-Escalation Techniques

Because the usual response to violence is a stress response (freeze, fight/ flight, fear), nonviolent crisis intervention and de-escalation tactics begin with self-awareness. To deal with the circumstance, the nurse must be able to control these reactions. The nurse must be able to spot warning signals of imminent conflict (clenched fists, and sudden change in tone of voice or body stance, and change in eye contact).

Restrictions on Physical Exercise

When alternative means of managing patient behavior have failed and there is a risk of injury to the patient or others, restraints are employed to restrict movement and activity. Violent (behavioral) and non-violent restraints are the two main types of restraints (clinical). The use of violent restraints is more widespread in psychiatric units or when people demonstrate hostile conduct. Nonviolent restrictions are more usually utilized to guarantee that the subject does not obstruct safe care.

Chemical Restraint

To manage an individual's behavior difficulties, chemical restraints involve the use of pharmaceutical sedatives. This sort of restriction should only be used when the patient's agitation or aggressiveness puts them or others in danger. Chemical constraints stop people from moving around, making their conduct more manageable.

Antipsychotic Medications

First-Generation

A range of first-generation antipsychotics is available, albeit their use is decreasing as atypical antipsychotic medicines become more widely available. Chlorpromazine (Thorazine®), Thioridazine hydrochloride (Mellaril®), Haloperidol (Haldol®), Pimozice (Orap®), Fluphenazine hydrochloride (Prolixin®), Molindone hydrochloride (Moban®), and Trifluoperazine hydrochloride (Stelazine®) are examples of first-generation antipsychotics.

Photosensitivity, sexual dysfunction, dry mouth, dry eyes, nasal congestion, blurred vision, constipation, urinary retention, exacerbation of narrow-angle glaucoma, dyskinesia, sedation, cognitive dulling, amenorrhea, menstrual irregularities, hyperglycemia or hypoglycemia, increased appetite, and weight gain are all possible side effects. Tics, lip-smacking, and eye blinking are the most prevalent extrapyramidal symptoms caused by antipsychotic drugs.

Second-Generation

Second-generation antipsychotics (SGAs), also known as atypical antipsychotics, include aripiprazole (Abilify®), clozapine (Clozaril®), olanzapine (Zyprexa®), quetiapine (Seroquel®), risperidone (Risperdal®), and ziprasidone (Geodon®) and are used to treat bipolar disorder, schizophrenia Females get more adverse effects than males, but the recommended doses are the same for both. Because researchers were concerned about teratogenic effects on fetuses, women were underrepresented in clinical trials of SGAs. Constipation, increased appetite, weight gain, urine retention, varied sexual side effects, increased prolactin, menstrual irregularities, increased diabetes risk, lowered blood pressure, dizziness, agranulocytosis, and leucopenia are all possible adverse effects.

Antidepressants

Depression is the most common reason for taking an antidepressant. Major depression, atypical depression, and anxiety disorders can all be added to this list.

SSRIs (selective serotonin reuptake inhibitors) stop serotonin from being reabsorbed at the presynaptic membrane. The amount of serotonin in the synapse for neurotransmission increases as a result of this. Antidepressants in this class have been found to alleviate depression and anxiety symptoms.

Tricyclic Antidepressants

Tricyclic antidepressants work by blocking muscarinic cholinergic receptors, histamine H1 receptors, and alpha1 noradrenergic receptors in addition to blocking serotonin and norepinephrine reuptake. Although these receptors do not influence depressive symptoms, their blocking has been linked to several of the tricyclics' adverse effects.

MAOIs

Monoamine oxidase inhibitors (MAOIs) have the same mechanism of action as their name suggests. These medications work by inhibiting the monoamine oxidase enzyme (MAO). MAO-A and MAO-B are two of these enzymes, and this type of drug suppresses both of them. Serotonin and norepinephrine are metabolized by these enzymes. Increased quantities of serotonin and norepinephrine are available for neurotransmission when these enzymes are inhibited.

Monoamine oxidase inhibitors (MAOIs) have side effects that are similar to antipsychotic drugs.

Anti-Anxiety Medications

Benzodiazepines

The most widely prescribed anxiety drugs are benzodiazepines. Chlordiazepoxide, lorazepam, diazepam, flurazepam, and triazolam are some of the most regularly prescribed. GABA, a neurotransmitter, is enhanced by benzodiazepines. This neurotransmitter slows the pace at which neurons fire, resulting in a reduction in anxiety sensations. The effect of sleepiness is one of the most common. Feelings of alienation, irritation, emotional lability, GI discomfort, dependence, or tolerance development are some of the other negative effects.

Practice Tests

Practice Test One

1. In an EKG, the P wave represents:

    A. Repolarization of the atria
    B. Depolarization of the ventricles
    C. Repolarization of the ventricles
    D. Depolarization of the atria

2. Which of the following findings indicates a positive Trousseau sign?

    A. The patient has twitching of their facial muscles when the area over the facial nerve is tapped
    B. When the patient's neck is flexed, they flex their hips and knees as well
    C. When the back of both hands are pressed together, almost hyperextending the wrists, there is a pain in the carpal tunnel region
    D. The patient has to twitch in their arm when a blood pressure cuff is left inflated on it for three minutes

3. Reliable and appropriate methods of evaluating aspiration risk for patients who are receiving enteral feedings (tube feedings) include all of the following except:

    A. Addition of blue dye to the formula to detect aspiration
    B. Monitor patient's management of oral secretions
    C. Monitor patient's level of consciousness
    D. Evaluate the patient's cough or gag reflex

4. Progesterone is secreted during the secretory phase of the menstrual cycle to help the implanted embryo and continue the pregnancy; it is secreted from a female's:

    A. Endoderm
    B. Anterior pituitary gland
    C. Mesoderm
    D. Corpus luteum

5. Which of the following is a type of malignancy of plasma cells in the bone marrow that leads to bone marrow failure and bone destruction?

A. Non-Hodgkin's lymphoma
B. Hodgkin's lymphoma
C. Myelodysplastic syndrome
D. Multiple myeloma

6. After change-of-shift report, which patient should the nurse assess first?

A. A 65-year-old patient with a recent surgical left leg amputation who is complaining of phantom pain
B. A 35-year-old patient with a fracture who is complaining that her new cast is tight
C. A 70-year-old patient with osteoporosis who is waiting for discharge
D. A 52-year-old patient with carpal tunnel syndrome complaining of pain

7. Clinical manifestations of tension pneumothorax may include:

A. Hypotension, distended neck veins, tracheal shift
B. Hypertension, absent breath sounds, distended neck veins
C. Hypo-resonance over pneumothorax, pallor, tachypnea
D. Hypo-resonance over pneumothorax, distended neck veins, tachycardia

8. Which of the following cardiac rhythms requires defibrillation?

A. Atrial fibrillation
B. Sinus tachycardia
C. Ventricular tachycardia
D. Asystole

9. In an adult patient with type 2 diabetes mellitus, the target goal for glycemic control is generally:

A. A1C < 8.0%
B. A1C < 6.5%

C. A1C < 7.0%
D. A1C < 7.5%

10. Which of the following statements is true related to serum albumin?

   A. It is a fasting laboratory test
   B. Persistent albuminuria is a reliable marker of poor nutritional status
   C. It is an indicator of the liver's ability to manufacture plasma proteins
   D. Normal values range from 1.5 to 3.5 g/dL

11. A patient you are caring for returns to the nursing unit following a py-elolithotomy for removal of stones in the kidney. A Penrose drain is in place. Which of the following actions would you include in the patient's postoperative plan of care?

   A. Weighing the dressings and adding the amount to the output
   B. Changing dressings frequently around the Penrose drain
   C. Irrigating the Penrose drain using sterile procedure
   D. Positioning the patient on the affected side

12. Which of the following statements is true related to autoimmune disorders?

   A. In autoimmune disorders, T cells produce autoantibodies (antibodies to host cells)
   B. In autoimmune disorders, B cells become autosensitized (sensitized to host cells)
   C. Idiopathic thrombocytopenic purpura (ITP) is a type of systemic autoimmune disease
   D. Autoimmune disorders occur when the immune system, failing to distinguish self from non-self, attacks its own body cells

13. The therapeutic drug level of phenytoin (Dilantin) is:

   A. 0.5-1 mcg/mL
   B. 5-10 mcg/mL
   C. 10-20 mcg/mL

D. 50-100 mcg/mL

14. A patient is asking the nurse a question regarding the purified protein derivative (PPD) intradermal test for tuberculosis. The nurse should base her response on the fact that:

    A. Skin testing does not differentiate between active and dormant tuberculosis infection
    B. Skin testing stimulates a reddened response in some patients and requires a second test be administered in 3 months
    C. The area of redness is measured in 3 days and determines whether tuberculosis is present
    D. The presence of a wheal at the injection site two days following PPD administration indicates active tuberculosis

15. Acute coronary syndrome is most often caused by:

    A. Hypovolemic shock
    B. Severe anemia
    C. Thrombus formation in narrowed coronary arteries
    D. Spasm of the smooth wall of the coronary arteries

16. All of the following statements are true related to urine ketone testing except:

    A. It is used to monitor for impending diabetic ketoacidosis
    B. It is generally recommended when blood glucose levels are consistently greater than 300 mg/dL
    C. It is recommended in the presence of hypoglycemia accompanied by diaphoresis, confusion, and slurred speech
    D. It primarily used in those with type 1 diabetes

17. The largest internal organ is the:

    A. Liver
    B. Colon
    C. Skin

D. Brain

18.   A woman is admitted to the hospital in active labor. In which of the following maternal conditions is a caesarean section delivery most likely to be indicated?

A. Gonorrhea
B. Endometriosis
C. Syphilis
D. Genital herpes outbreak

19.   The physician has ordered diphenhydramine hydrochloride (Benadryl) 50 mg PO for a patient with allergies. The nurse is aware this medication administered PO will reach its peak effect how long after administration?

A. 30-60 minutes
B. 1-4 hours
C. 15-20 minutes
D. 4-7 hours

20.   What reflex grade would be assigned to a patient with a hypoactive patellar reflex?

A. Grade 3+
B. Grade 0
C. Grade 1+
D. Grade 2+

21.   A mixture of blood and pleural fluid accumulating in the pleural space that restricts lung expansion is known as:

A. Hemorrhagic pleural effusion
B. Empyema
C. Chylothorax
D. Hemothorax

22. Which of the following is an endogenous chemical that is released in response to excessive stretching of the heart muscle cells?

   A. Myoglobin
   B. Brain natriuretic peptide (BNP)
   C. Troponin
   D. Creatinine phosphokinase (CPK)

23. Type 2 diabetes mellitus (DM) accounts for what percentage of the DM population globally?

   A. 60%
   B. 70%
   C. 80%
   D. 90%

24. You are caring for a patient with cirrhosis (chronic liver damage) and are aware that symptoms of portal hypertension are caused by:

   A. Degeneration of Kupffer cells
   B. Infection of the liver
   C. Blockage in the cystic and hepatic ducts
   D. Blockage of blood flow in the portal vein

25. Your patient has a diagnosis of benign prostatic hypertrophy (BPH) and is scheduled for a transurethral resection of the prostate (TURP). When providing preoperative teaching, all of the following points are appropriate to include except:

   A. TURP is the most common operation for BPH
   B. The purpose and function of an indwelling urinary catheter
   C. He will be pain-free after surgery
   D. Bladder spasms may occur

26. Which immunoglobulin is the only maternal antibody that crosses the placenta?

    A. IgA
    B. IgD
    C. IgG
    D. IgM

27. Which of the following is not a risk factor for a hemorrhagic stroke?

    A. Administration of tPA
    B. Anticoagulant use
    C. Head trauma
    D. Chronic hypotension

28. To maximize the benefit of therapy, continuous passive motion (CPM) should be used how frequently?

    A. At least 6-8 hours daily
    B. At least three times per week
    C. At least 10 hours per day
    D. At least once daily

29. You are caring for a patient who was admitted with heart failure who appears to be in respiratory distress and has an O2 sat of 83%. Upon placing a non-rebreather, the patient's O2 sat increases to and sustains 92%, and the patient's symptoms seem less severe. Which of the following considerations should direct your continued care?

    A. The patient's O2 sat is not responding as it should, and more advanced respiratory treatment is necessary
    B. The flow rate to the non-rebreather should be increased until the patient has an O2 sat of at least 95%
    C. The patient has responded appropriately to treatment, but should be monitored for potential changes
    D. The patient is not likely to survive the dyspnea that they are experiencing

30. You are completing the admission assessment on a male patient whose admitting diagnosis includes a history of cardiac disease. Upon auscultation you should:

A. Ask the patient to take deep breaths when listening for carotid bruits
B. Recognize bruits as abnormal swishing sounds caused by abnormal blood flow patterns or incompetent valves when you listen to the patient's heart sounds
C. Recognize bruits as low-frequency vibrations caused by inflamed, infected or damaged tissues
D. Ask the patient to hold his breath when listening for carotid bruits

31. Antidiuretic hormone (ADH) is synthesized in the:

A. Hypothalamus
B. Pineal gland
C. Pituitary gland
D. Thalamus

32. When changing your patient's ileostomy bag, you notice that the peristomal skin is irritated. Which of these actions would be the most appropriate before reapplying the appliance?

A. Clean the site with betadine solution
B. Wash the area with soap and water
C. Use a solid skin barrier
D. Request an order for a topical antibiotic

33. Decreased glomerular filtration rate (GFR) results in which of the following?

A. Increased filtering of creatinine resulting in decreased serum creatinine levels
B. Increased filtering of creatinine resulting in increased serum creatinine levels
C. Decreased filtering of creatinine resulting in decreased serum creatinine levels

D. Decreased filtering of creatinine resulting in increased serum creatinine levels

34. Which of the following four patients has the greatest risk of developing a healthcare associated infection (HAI)?

    A. An 89-year-old male who was is being admitted today from home for failure to thrive and who has early signs of pneumonia
    B. A 53-year-old male who was transferred from the ICU and was extubated four days ago
    C. A 73-year-old female who has an IV and is scheduled for a head CT after a ground-level fall
    D. An 84-year-old female who is being admitted today from a nursing home with a change in mental status and who has a catheter that was placed 12 days ago

35. Supination is defined as:

    A. Turning a part away from midline
    B. Turning a part toward midline
    C. Turning upward
    D. Turning downward

36. Which of the following respiratory conditions is not known to be caused by a SARS-CoV-2 infection?

    A. Acute respiratory distress syndrome (ARDS)
    B. Pneumonia
    C. Pulmonary embolism
    D. Emphysema

37. A 62-year-old male patient with a recent history of rheumatic fever is admitted to the medical-surgical unit with the following symptoms:

    - Subjective: Shortness of breath, chest pain, syncope
    - Objective: Peripheral edema, neck vein distension, weight gain, cyanosis, hepatomegaly, bounding pulses, cardiac arrhythmia

Which of the following is most likely this patient's primary diagnosis?

    A. Left heart failure
    B. Aortic valve stenosis
    C. Endocarditis
    D. Abdominal aortic aneurysm

38.   All of the following statement are true related to hyperosmolar hypergly-cemic syndrome (HHS) except:

    A. Ketosis may be only slight or may be absent in this condition
    B. It is characterized by severe dehydration
    C. Its onset occurs more rapidly than diabetic ketoacidosis
    D. Stupor and coma are common neurological symptoms of this condition

39.   Your patient, Mrs. Y., is scheduled for an oral cholecystogram. You in-struct her that:

    A. Radiopaque dye will be injected during the procedure
    B. She may be asked to drink milk prior to or during the procedure
    C. She may be asked to eat a piece of fried chicken for the procedure
    D. She may be asked to drink barium for the procedure

40.   What is the primary function of the kidneys?

    A. To synthesize the hormones erythropoietin, vitamin D, renal prosta-glandins, and renin
    B. To detoxify the blood
    C. To eliminate wastes
    D. To maintain a stable internal environment for optimal cell and tissue metabolism

41.   You are providing a transfusion to a patient with pernicious anemia when they report that they suddenly feel short of breath. Which of the follow-ing interventions is most important?

    A. Administer oxygen

B. Stop the transfusion
C. Notify the doctor
D. Assess the patient's lung sounds

42. You are teaching a newly diagnosed patient with osteoporosis about strategies to prevent falls. All of these points should be included except:

    A. Exercise will help build your strength, but you should rest when you are tired
    B. Remove throw rugs and other obstacles at home
    C. You should expect a few bumps and bruises when you go home
    D. Wear a hip protector when ambulating

43. You are supervising a new nurse who is caring for a patient with lung cancer. Which of the following statements by the new nurse would require correction?

    A. "Lung cancer is the most common respiratory complication caused by smoking."
    B. "Small-cell carcinoma is an aggressive type of lung cancer that spreads quickly."
    C. "Lung cancer is the most common type of cancer worldwide."
    D. "Smoking makes your risk of developing lung cancer about ten times greater."

44. When discharging a patient who was recently diagnosed with coronary artery disease, which of the following statements by the patient indicates that further teaching is needed?

    A. "If I am more active, my risks from coronary artery disease will be lower."
    B. "Getting older is not something I can control, but it won't make my risk of coronary artery disease worse."
    C. "Smoking is something I can control. If I stop smoking, I will reduce the risks of coronary artery disease."
    D. "Low blood pressure doesn't raise my risk of coronary artery disease."

45. The physician has ordered a 24-hour urine test for metanephrine on a patient. This test is used in the diagnosis of which of the following conditions?

   A. Pheochromocytomas
   B. Addison's disease
   C. Diabetes mellitus
   D. Diabetes insipidus

46. A patient is scheduled for a closed liver biopsy. Nursing responsibilities related to this procedure include all of the following except:

   A. Monitoring the large incision for signs of bleeding
   B. Obtaining informed consent
   C. Monitoring for indications of respiratory distress following the procedure
   D. Maintaining the patient on flat bed rest or positioned on the right side for 24 hours after the procedure

47. Which of the following patients would be the best candidate for a condom catheter?

   A. A 72-year-old female who has functional incontinence and rheumatoid arthritis
   B. A 53-year-old male with stress incontinence who is scheduled for an IV pyelogram
   C. A 62-year-old male with gout and difficulty urinating due to benign prostatic hyperplasia (BPH)
   D. A 87-year-old male with advanced dementia and urge incontinence

48. Which of the following blood components is decreased in anemia?

   A. Granulocytes
   B. Platelets
   C. Erythrocytes
   D. Leukocytes

49. All of the following medications are sodium channel blockers except:

    A. Lamotrigine (Lamictal)
    B. Carbamazepine (Tegretol)
    C. Clonazepam (Klonopin)
    D. Phenytoin (Dilantin)

50. The most common type of lung cancer is:

    A. Small cell lung cancer
    B. Adenocarcinomas
    C. Squamous cell cancer
    D. Large cell cancer

51. A pregnant woman may have which of the following heart sounds upon auscultation?

    A. A split S2 heart sound
    B. S3 heart sound
    C. A pericardial knock
    D. S4 heart sound

52. An obese, type 2 diabetic patient who is non-insulin dependent is best controlled by weight loss for which of the following reasons?

    A. Because obesity reduces insulin binding at receptor sites
    B. Because obesity reduces the number of insulin receptors
    C. Because obesity reduces pancreatic islet cell exhaustion
    D. Because obesity reduces pancreatic insulin production

53. You are admitting a 54-year-old female who came to the ER for changes in mental status. Upon assessment, you note ascites, icterus, and confusion. The patient has a history of GERD, alcoholism, asthma, and atrial fibrillation. Which of the following is most likely the cause of the patient's confusion?

    A. Elevated ammonia levels

B. Fluid in the lungs, causing hypoxia

C. Thrombosis in the brain

D. Inflammation of the airways, causing hypoxia

54. A vaginal infection characterized by discharge that is thin, greenish-yellow or gray, and bubbly is most likely:

A. Vulvovaginal candidiasis

B. Trichomoniasis vaginitis

C. Dyspareunia

D. Bacterial vaginosis

55. As a nurse on an adult medical-surgical floor, which type of leukemia are you least likely to encounter?

A. Acute lymphoblastic leukemia (ALL)

B. Chronic myelogenous leukemia (CML)

C. Chronic lymphocytic leukemia (CLL)

D. Acute myelogenous leukemia (AML)

56. You are caring for a patient who has just been diagnosed with Guillain-Barré Syndrome. Which statement made by the patient is incorrect?

A. "Most people are not likely to survive Guillain-Barré Syndrome."

B. "Guillain-Barré Syndrome is caused because my immune system is attacking my nerves."

C. "Guillain-Barré Syndrome can eventually completely resolve."

D. "I may need to have a machine breathe for me."

57. A patient with which of the following conditions would be most likely to be found sitting on the side of the bed, leaning forward, with an anxious expression?

A. Chronic bronchitis

B. Pleural effusion

C. Emphysema

D. Gastroesophageal reflux disease

58.	Which of the following medications is not indicated for a patient who is experiencing hypertension?

A. Norepinephrine (Levophed)
B. Olmesartan (Benicar)
C. Enalapril (Vasotec)
D. Carvedilol (Coreg)

59.	Diagnostic tests for primary hyperparathyroidism include all of the following except:

A. Evidence of bone resorption on radiography and bone scan
B. Elevated serum calcium and parathyroid hormone
C. Urinary potassium concentration
D. Evidence of kidney stones

60.	Factors that may play a role in the development of peptic ulcer disease include all of the following except:

A. The chronic use of aspirin
B. The inflammation of mucosa due to *H. pylori*
C. Cigarette smoking
D. Decreased hydrochloric acid production in the stomach

61.	This renal hormone stimulates bone marrow production of red blood cells (RBCs):

A. Prostaglandins
B. Vitamin D
C. Renin
D. Erythropoietin

62.	Which of the following is an early sign of systemic lupus erythematosus (SLE)?

A. Joint pain
B. Kidney failure

C. Cardiac dysrhythmias

D. Restrictive lung disease

63. This part of the central nervous system is located in the brainstem. It participates in control of the respiratory and gastrointestinal function. It is known as the:

A. Pia mater

B. Medulla

C. Dura mater

D. Reticular activating system

64. You are assessing a patient's lung sounds and note bronchovesicular wheezing on expiration. Which of the following conditions is this type of breath sound most likely to be associated with?

A. Heart failure

B. Anaphylaxis

C. Asthma

D. Pneumonia

65. The volume of blood pumped from the ventricle during one heartbeat is known as:

A. Cardiac output

B. Pulse pressure

C. Stroke volume

D. Preload

66. Which of the following is true about diabetic neuropathy?

A. Diabetic neuropathy can be prevented by wearing loose socks and keeping the legs elevated

B. Diabetic neuropathy is one of the contributing factors to diabetes-related amputations

C. Diabetic neuropathy is an uncommon complication of diabetes mellitus

D. Diabetic neuropathy is reversible in some cases

67. Which of the following pharmacotherapeutic agents used to treat gastrointestinal disorders can cause gastrointestinal infections if taken long-term?

    A. Gastric mucosal protectants
    B. Antiemetics
    C. Antacids
    D. Proton pump inhibitors

68. A patient is frustrated and embarrassed by urinary incontinence. Which of the following measures should the nurse include in a bladder retraining program?

    A. Assessing present elimination patterns
    B. Restricting fluid intake to reduce the need to void
    C. Establishing a predetermined fluid intake pattern for the patient
    D. Encouraging the patient to increase the time between voidings

69. Which of the follow interventions would be least helpful for preventing infection in a patient with neutropenia?

    A. Following best practices for hand hygiene
    B. Instructing the patient to bathe and perform oral care regularly
    C. Only allowing visitors who may be sick to spend two minutes or less with the patient
    D. Not allowing fresh fruits of vegetables into the patient's room

70. The most common form of joint disease is:

    A. Scoliosis
    B. Fibromyalgia
    C. Rheumatoid arthritis
    D. Osteoarthritis

71. Of the following factors, which might alter the result of pulse oximetry?

    A. The patient's age, patient movement, acrylic nails

B. Patient's age, hypervolemia, patient movement

C. The patient's skin color, hypovolemia, temperature of appendage

D. Hypervolemia, the patient's skin color, acrylic nails

72. You are admitting a 45-year-old male who presented to the emergency room because his doctor sent him with "abnormal vital signs." The patient has BP 98/59, HR 34, Temp 98.7, RR 14, and O2 sat 98% on room air. The patient's doctor sent an EKG performed today showing sinus bradycardia. The patient is alert, oriented, and denies any symptoms. Which of the following interventions is most important?

A. Administer atropine 0.5mg IV STAT

B. Administer 1L NS bolus

C. Continue to monitor the patient

D. Prepare for transcutaneous pacing

73. When testing plasma glucose levels in the adult patient with diabetes, postprandial levels should be obtained when?

A. 1-2 hours after the beginning of the meal

B. 2-3 hours after the end of the meal

C. 1-2 hours before the meal

D. 2-3 hours after the beginning of the meal

74. Which of the following is the least important educational point for a patient about to undergo a endoscopy?

A. The length of the procedure

B. What to expect during the procedure

C. Preparation required prior to procedure

D. The purpose of the procedure

75. In the ischemic phase of the menstrual cycle, estrogen and progesterone levels fall due to:

A. Endometrial thickening

B. A decrease in follicle stimulating hormone from the anterior pituitary gland

C. Corpus luteum formation

D. Degeneration of the corpus luteum

76. When human immunodeficiency virus (HIV) initially attaches to a host cell, what genetic material is released into the cell's cytoplasm?

A. RNA

B. DNA

C. Chromosome

D. Ribosome

77. You are caring for a patient who suddenly develops unilateral weakness. Which of the following interventions should be performed first?

A. CT scan

B. Assess the patient's NIH stroke scale

C. Check the patient's blood glucose level

D. Administer tPA

78. Which type of pneumothorax occurs when air has been drawn into the pleural space and is unable to escape, thus causing a build up of pressure and resulting in compression of all structures within the thorax?

A. Traumatic pneumothorax

B. Inflation pneumothorax

C. Tension pneumothorax

D. Spontaneous pneumothorax

79. This chamber of the heart is much thicker than the others because it pumps blood to the entire body:

A. Left ventricle

B. Right ventricle

C. Right atrium

D. Left atrium

80. Which of the following insulins can be administered intravenously?

    A. Rapid-acting insulin
    B. Regular insulin
    C. All types of insulin can be administered intravenously
    D. Long-acting insulin

81. What amount of upper GI tract blood loss would be defined as "acute" or "massive" in adults?

    A. 500 mL
    B. 1500 mL
    C. 1000 mL
    D. 800 mL

82. You are caring for a patient with chronic kidney disease who asks you how peritoneal dialysis works. Which response is most correct?

    A. "A hypertonic solution containing heparin will be instilled into your abdomen and left there for several hours."
    B. "Peritoneal dialysis will usually only need to be done three days a week."
    C. "Peritoneal dialysis can be performed at home, but will require a nurse to set it up each time."
    D. "You will need a tube that is surgically inserted into the space between your intestines and the wall of your abdomen."

83. A freckle is an example of which of the following types of lesions?

    A. Pustule
    B. Macule
    C. Papule
    D. Patch

84.   A patient with an open fracture of the radius has a plaster cast applied in the emergency department. The nurse provides home-care instructions and tells the patient to seek medical attention if which of the following occurs?

A. Numbness and tingling are felt in the fingers
B. Scant bloody drainage is noted in the cast during the first 6 hours after application
C. The entire cast feels warm during the first 24 hours after application
D. The cast feels heavy and damp 24 hours after application

85.   The adenoids are located on the posterior wall of the:

A. Laryngopharynx
B. Nasopharynx
C. Oropharynx
D. Cricoid cartilage

86.   You are starting your shift and receive report on the following four patients. Which patient should you see first?

A. A patient who is on comfort care measures who is expected to pass at any time
B. A patient who has a MAP that has decreased from 84 to 70
C. A patient who recently received a sublingual nitroglycerin and says that his chest pain turned into a headache
D. A patient with hypokalemia who had a run of ventricular tachycardia that resolved by itself

87.   All of the following statements related to carbohydrate intake in the diabetic patient are true except:

A. Scientific evidence does not support the restriction of sucrose
B. Daily carbohydrate intake depends on blood glucose and lipid goals
C. Low-carbohydrate diets, which restrict total carbohydrates to less than 130 g/day, are recommended in the management of diabetes mellitus
D. Fiber intake should be 25-35 g/day

88. Which of the following medications promotes the absorption of fluids into stool, increasing the bulk of stools, which stimulates peristalsis?

    A. Docusate (Colace)
    B. Psyllium (Metamucil)
    C. Mineral oil
    D. Bisacodyl (Dulcolax)

89. You are providing teaching to a patient who is about to have a transurethral resection of the prostate (TURP). Which of the following statements indicates that further teaching is needed?

    A. "I will not be able to have intercourse after this surgery."
    B. "I will probably go home with a catheter after this surgery."
    C. "If I notice blood in my urine after the surgery, this is normal."
    D. "I may need to take medications for bladder spasms after my surgery."

90. You are caring for a patient who was just diagnosed with Hodgkin's lymphoma who asks you "What are my chances of surviving this cancer?" Which of the following responses is best?

    A. "Your odds of surviving would be better if you had non-Hodgkin's lymphoma."
    B. "Hodgkin's lymphoma is one of the most treatable cancers an adult can have."
    C. "Hodgkin's lymphoma is not something that can kill you; you will just be sick for a few months."
    D. "There is no cure for Hodgkin's lymphoma, and it is almost always a terminal disease."

91. A patient you are caring for is on day one post-op following a right total knee arthroplasty (TKA) and develops symptoms of compartment syndrome. Which of the following nursing interventions is indicated?

    A. Elevate the patient's right lower extremity above heart level
    B. Apply TED hose to control peripheral edema
    C. Keep the patient's right lower extremity at heart level

D. Obtain a specimen of incisional drainage for culture and sensitivity

92. A patient is coughing up sputum with a musty odor that is bluish-green in color. The nurse suspects which of the following conditions?

    A. Pneumococcal pneumonia
    B. Pseudomonas pneumonia
    C. Serratia pneumonia
    D. Klebsiella pneumonia

93. Which of the following patient complaints should be addressed first?

    A. A 32-year-old female who complains of a new "fluttering" sensation in her chest that started five minutes ago
    B. A 72-year-old female who complains of a headache and has a blood pressure of 189/101
    C. A 68-year-old male with heart failure who is struggling to breathe
    D. A 54-year-old male complaining of crushing chest pain

94. Primary adrenocortical hypofunction involving destruction of the adrenal cortex is known as:

    A. Addison's disease
    B. Adrenal Cushing's syndrome
    C. Ectopic Cushing's syndrome
    D. Pituitary Cushing's disease

95. A gastric emptying study is an example of which of the following?

    A. Ultrasonography
    B. A computerized tomography (CT) scan
    C. Endoscopy
    D. A nuclear imaging scan

96. Which of the following causes of acute kidney injury is considered a cause of pre-renal acute kidney injury (AKI)?

   A. Acute tubular necrosis
   B. Hemorrhagic shock
   C. Renal calculi
   D. Post-infectious glomerulonephritis

97. Which of the following findings in a patient who has immune thrombocytopenia purpura requires immediate further assessment?

   A. Dry and tender gums that are sore when eating
   B. Urine that is an amber color
   C. Excessive itchiness on the palms of the hands and soles of the feet
   D. A rash that consists of tiny, pinpoint, flat red spots

98. The mnemonic device, "R-I-C-E," is used to describe the treatment of choice for any acute musculoskeletal injury. What do the letters stand for?

   A. Relax, Inhibit, Control, Execute
   B. Relax, Ice, Contain, Elevate
   C. Rest, Ice, Compress, Elevate
   D. Rest, Ice, Contract , Elevate

99. A 38-year-old patient is admitted to the hospital with the following clinical manifestations: dyspnea, tachypnea, and pink, frothy sputum. The nurse determines that the patient is experiencing:

   A. Lung cancer
   B. Pulmonary embolism
   C. Pleural effusion
   D. Lung abscess

100. The most critical period following an acute myocardial infarction (MI) is within the:

   A. First 24 to 48 hours

B. First 30 to 60 minutes

C. First 6 to 24 hours

D. First 2 to 4 hours

101. You are caring for a patient with Grave's disease. Which of the following statements made by the patient indicate their understanding of the disease process?

A. "My heart is likely to beat more slowly than most peoples'."

B. "My eyes may stick out more because of this disease."

C. "I should increase my intake of foods containing iodine."

D. "It is very important that I do not miss doses of my blood thinning medication when treating this disease."

102. Which type of hepatitis virus is spread through the fecal/oral route?

A. Hepatitis B (HVB)

B. Hepatitis A (HVA)

C. Hepatitis C (HVC)

D. Hepatitis G (HVG)

103. Which of the following statements is true about performing a urinalysis on a patient with suspected kidney stones?

A. A urinalysis will not give any helpful information related to the presence of kidney stones

B. A urinalysis may show blood in the urine that indicates a kidney stone may be present

C. A urinalysis will show the presence of minerals that can indicate a kidney stone may be present

D. A urinalysis can show white blood cells that may indicate inflammation caused by kidney stones

104. A patient's burn wound has been covered with an allograft. The nurse is aware that an allograft is:

A. Skin from the same species donor

B. Artificial skin

C. A graft that is transferred from one location to another on the same individual

D. Skin from a different species donor

105. Which of the following diagnostic studies is considered the "gold standard" for diagnosing osteoporosis?

A. X-ray

B. CT scan

C. MRI

D. DEXA

106. You are reviewing documentation on a patient in your care, and you see that rhonchi lung sounds were present on the previous shift. Upon chest auscultation, you note that rhonchi are still present in your patient. You are aware that:

A. Rhonchi are caused by inflamed surfaces of the pleural membranes moving against each other

B. Rhonchi are an expiratory sound caused by bronchial narrowing due to inflammation, fluid, or obstruction

C. Rhonchi are audible without a stethoscope

D. Rhonchi are most commonly heard on inspiration and are caused by upper airway obstruction

107. This non-specific enzyme found in the heart and skeletal muscle is released into the bloodstream with myocardial damage, rising 30 minutes to 2 hours after onset of myocardial infarction (MI). What is it?

A. Myoglobin

B. Brain natriuretic peptide (BNP)

C. Troponin

D. Creatinine phosphokinase (CPK)

108. All of the following are examples of rapid-acting insulin except:

A. NPH (Humulin N)
B. Lispro (Humalog)
C. Glulisine (Apidra)
D. Aspart (Novolog)

109. All of the following statements are true related to duodenal ulcers except:

A. Duodenal ulcers result from increased production of HCL in the stomach due to rapid emptying of stomach contents
B. There is a correlation between duodenal ulcers and NSAID use
C. Patients present with decreased appetite and weight loss
D. Duodenal ulcers account for 80% of all peptic ulcers

110. In a patient with glomerulonephritis, an acute inflammation of the kidney, the nurse could anticipate all of the following laboratory findings except:

A. Hematuria
B. Proteinuria
C. Decreased sedimentation rate
D. Positive antibody test for streptokinase exoenzymes

111. Which of the following diagnostic antibody tests is the most common confirmatory test for HIV?

A. Western blot
B. Rapid HIV antibody test
C. Indirect immunofluorescence assay
D. Enzyme immunoassay test

112. Which of the following are mature bone cells that deliver oxygen and nutrition, and remove wastes to maintain bone health?

A. Osteophytes
B. Osteoclasts
C. Osteoblasts

D. Osteocytes

113. A nurse performs an admission assessment on a patient with a diagnosis of active tuberculosis. The nurse reviews the result of which diagnostic test that will confirm this diagnosis?

    A. Chest x-ray
    B. Tuberculin skin test
    C. Bronchoscopy
    D. Sputum culture

114. While you are precepting a new nurse, which of the following statements by the new nurse indicates that he understands your teaching?

    A. "Angina is primarily chest pain, but in about 25% of cases, it radiates into the low back and upper legs."
    B. "Another name for angina is myocardial infarction."
    C. "If a patient is experiencing angina, we should have the crash cart by their bedside."
    D. "Prinzmetal's angina is not caused by hardening of the arteries in the heart."

115. Which of the following is true about pheochromocytomas?

    A. Surgery on these tumors is often very successful
    B. These tumors often secrete hormones that stimulate the parasympathetic system
    C. These tumors most often metastasize extensively before they are found
    D. Hypoglycemia is a common symptom of these tumors

116. Which of the following would not change with a severe acute GI bleed that started 15 minutes ago?

    A. Heart rate
    B. Hemoglobin
    C. Blood pressure
    D. Skin color and quality

117. A disorder characterized by the formation of grape-like clusters of fluid-filled cysts that replace normal kidney tissue is:

    A. Proliferative glomerulonephritis
    B. Interstitial cystitis
    C. Diffuse glomerulonephritis
    D. Polycystic kidney disease

118. The epidermis on the palms of the hands and soles of the feet is composed of how many layers?

    A. Five
    B. Four
    C. Three
    D. Two

119. All of the following statements related to Myasthenia Gravis (MG) are true except:

    A. Most common muscles involved are respiratory muscles
    B. It worsens with exercise and improves with rest
    C. It is an acquired autoimmune disease
    D. Onset may occur at any age

120. Which of the following is a long-acting beta-adrenergic agonist administered by inhalation and used for long-term control (not short-term or rescue relief) of bronchospasm?

    A. Albuterol (Proventil, Ventolin)
    B. Bitolterol (Tornalate)
    C. Salmeterol (Serevent)
    D. Levalbuterol (Xopenex)

121. The most common type of cardiomyopathy is:

    A. Bacterial
    B. Restrictive

C. Hypertrophic

D. Dilated

122. You are caring for a female patient with Cushing's syndrome. You know that treatment is successful when there is a decline in:

A. Bone mineralization

B. Hair loss

C. Menstrual flow

D. Serum glucose levels

123. Which of the following statements related to chronic liver failure is true?

A. The course of chronic liver disease is approximately 8 to 26 weeks

B. Ascites causes the abdomen to become enlarged and can result in severe respiratory distress

C. The usual cause is drug toxicity (acetaminophen)

D. Encephalopathy represents early-stage liver disease

124. The nurse is caring for a patient with acute kidney failure, and during the shift, the patient becomes more confused and irritable. The nurse understands that the most likely cause of the change in behavior is due to:

A. Hyperkalemia

B. Dehydration

C. Elevated blood urea nitrogen (BUN)

D. Hypernatremia

125. The presence of the Philadelphia chromosome is definitive for the diagnosis of which of the following leukemias?

A. Chronic myelogenous leukemia (CML)

B. Chronic lymphocytic leukemia (CLL)

C. Acute myelogenous leukemia (AML)

D. Acute lymphocytic leukemia (ALL)

126. A patient who is lying supine in bed complains of pain during range of motion exercises when he points his toes toward the foot of the bed. What is this type of joint movement called?

    A. Dorsiflexion
    B. Plantarflexion
    C. Circumduction
    D. Eversion

127. You are caring for a patient whose ABG shows an PaO2 of 80. A nursing student asks you what this means. Which response is the best?

    A. "The patient is quite hypoxic, and we should place him on oxygen immediately."
    B. "We need to look at the patient's pH to fully understand what this value means."
    C. "This patient's PaO2 is normal."
    D. "This patient will require intubation."

128. A 82-year-old female complains of sudden pain between her shoulder blades. Which of the following ordered tests should be performed first?

    A. Cardiac catheterization
    B. MRI
    C. EKG
    D. CT of the cervical and thoracic spine

129. All of the following statements are true related to the parathyroid except:

    A. It consists of two lobes joined by a thin isthmus
    B. It is essential for calcium regulation
    C. It is responsible for secreting parathyroid hormone
    D. It is located close to, or embedded in, the posterior portion of the thyroid

130. All of the following statements related to esophageal narrowing are true except:

    A. The patient may experience substernal chest pain associated with meals
    B. The condition is not gender or age specific
    C. Painful swallowing occurs early in the condition
    D. The inability to belch is a sign that the disease has progressed

131. All of the following conditions have been linked to the development of malignant ovarian tumors except:

    A. High-fat diet
    B. Endometriosis
    C. Celibacy
    D. Multiple pregnancies

132. You are caring for a male patient with severe psoriasis. When inspecting his affected areas, you expect to see which type of secondary lesions?

    A. Cysts
    B. Ulcers
    C. Scales
    D. Crusts

133. All of the following statements related to rheumatoid arthritis (RA) are true except:

    A. RA is the most common articular disease in adults
    B. Isometric exercises are used in RA patients to preserve and improve muscle function
    C. Disease-modifying anti-rheumatic drugs (DMARDs) should be initiated early in RA treatment
    D. No single set of tests can confirm diagnosis of RA

134. Pneumonia that involves an entire lobe of the lung is classified as:

    A. Lobar pneumonia
    B. Bronchopneumonia
    C. Interstitial pneumonia
    D. Legionnaires pneumonia

135. Which of the following medications is most likely to cause angioedema?

    A. Valsartan (Diovan)
    B. Diltiazem (Cardizem)
    C. Nadolol (Corgard)
    D. Captopril (Capoten)

136. The hemoglobin A1C level indicates a patient's blood glucose control over which of the following (approximate) times?

    A. The previous 30 days
    B. The previous 3 weeks
    C. The previous 3 days
    D. The previous 3 months

137. Of the following menus, which is the most appropriate for a patient with diarrhea?

    A. Jello, fish, milk
    B. Coffee, noodles, fish
    C. Bananas, fried chicken, mashed potatoes
    D. Cooked carrots, bananas, potatoes

138. A patient who is being treated for kidney stones asks you what he can do to reduce his risk of kidney stones in the future. Which of the following responses is least correct?

    A. "Avoid foods that contain calcium, oxalates, and purines."
    B. "Stay as active as you can and exercise regularly."
    C. "Drink plenty of water and avoid sugary or caffeinated drinks."

D. "Be sure to empty your bladder more frequently."

139. The nurse is preparing to teach a patient with iron deficiency anemia about the diet to follow after hospital discharge. Which of the following foods should be included in the diet?

A. Eggs
B. Lettuce
C. Legumes
D. Cheese

140. Lordosis is defined as:

A. Posterior concavity of the sacral spine
B. Posterior concavity of the lumbar spine
C. Greater than 45-degree curvature of thoracic spine
D. Lateral curvature of the spine

141. A patient is scheduled for pulmonary function testing. Prior to the test, it is the nurse's responsibility to:

A. Obtain the patient's weight only
B. Administer all oral and inhaled medications as ordered to ensure accuracy of the tests
C. Make sure the comatose patient's family has signed the proper consent forms
D. Notify the physician if the patient is confused and unable to follow directions

142. Which of the following is true when hypertension is diagnosed?

A. A diagnosis of hypertension must take the patient's BMI into consideration
B. Hypertension must be diagnosed by using blood pressure readings from at least two different patient visits or occasions
C. If only the first number of the blood pressure is elevated, the patient will likely be specifically diagnosed with systolic hypertension

D. Secondary hypertension is often due to excessive sodium intake

143. The syndrome of inappropriate antidiuretic hormone (SIADH) is:

    A. Characterized by decreased renal responsiveness to antidiuretic hormone
    B. Characterized by hypernatremia
    C. Characterized by excessive release of antidiuretic hormone
    D. Characterized by the suppression of antidiuretic hormone

144. You are establishing priorities for morning assessments of your patients. Which of the following patients should you assess first?

    A. The newly admitted patient with acute abdominal pain
    B. The sleeping patient who received pain medication 1 hour ago
    C. The patient who needs an abdominal dressing changed (postoperative day 3)
    D. The patient receiving continuous tube feedings who needs the residual checked

145. A 65-year-old patient with benign prostatic hypertrophy (BPH) doesn't respond to medical treatment and is admitted to the facility for prostate gland surgery. Before providing preoperative and postoperative instructions to the patient, the nurse asks the surgeon which prostatectomy procedure will be performed.
    • What is the most widely used surgical procedure for BPH treatment?

    A. Suprapubic prostatectomy
    B. Retropubic prostatectomy
    C. Transurethral resection of prostate (TURP)
    D. Transurethral incision of the prostate

146. While completing the admission assessment of a patient who is non-ambulatory and is unable to move or reposition himself in bed, you note an intact blood-filled blister on the heel. You should document this wound as which of the following?

    A. Unstageable pressure ulcer
    B. Stage II pressure ulcer
    C. Suspected deep tissue injury
    D. Stage I pressure ulcer

147. A Colles' fracture is most likely to be diagnosed in which of the following patients?

    A. An elderly woman who has fallen out of bed whose right leg is externally rotated and shorter than the left
    B. A teenage girl who was hit by another player during a soccer game who reports extreme pain in her left ankle
    C. A 98-pound male patient with lung cancer, complaining of pain in his right rib area
    D. A young boy who has slipped on the ice and is complaining of severe pain in his wrist

148. You are administering medications to a patient who has asthma. Which of the following is true?

    A. Inhaled bronchodilators should be administered before inhaled steroids
    B. Oral steroids should be administered before inhaled bronchodilators
    C. Routine inhaled bronchodilators do not need be administered at all unless the patient shows signs of respiratory distress
    D. Inhaled steroids should be administered before inhaled bronchodilators

149. What is Levine's sign?

    A. A universal sign of acute appendicitis
    B. A universal sign of choking
    C. A universal sign of a deep vein thrombosis
    D. A universal sign of coronary artery disease

150. Which of the following patients would be most at risk for developing diabetes insipidus?

    A. A 54-year-old male with a family history of syndrome of inappropriate antidiuretic hormone secretion (SIADH)
    B. A 32-year-old female with brain cancer that is inoperable
    C. A 27-year-old female who is prediabetic and is now 8 weeks pregnant
    D. A 92-year-old male with end stage renal disease

Answer Key

Q.	1	2	3	4	5	6	7	8	9	10	11	12	13	14	15
A.	D	D	A	D	D	A	A	C	C	C	B	D	C	A	C

Q.	16	17	18	19	20	21	22	23	24	25	26	27	28	29	30
A.	C	A	D	B	C	A	B	D	D	C	C	D	A	A	D

Q.	31	32	33	34	35	36	37	38	39	40	41	42	43	44	45
A.	A	C	D	D	C	D	B	C	B	D	B	C	A	B	A

Q.	46	47	48	49	50	51	52	53	57	55	56	57	58	59	60
A.	A	B	C	C	B	B	A	A	B	A	A	C	A	C	D

Q.	61	62	63	64	65	66	67	68	69	70	71	72	73	74	75
A.	D	A	B	C	C	B	D	A	C	D	C	C	A	A	D

Q.	76	77	78	79	80	81	82	83	84	85	86	87	88	89	90
A.	A	A	C	A	B	B	D	B	A	B	D	C	B	A	B

Q.	91	92	93	94	95	96	97	98	99	100	101	102	103	104	105
A.	C	B	C	A	D	B	D	C	B	C	B	B	B	A	D

Q.	106	107	108	109	110	111	112	113	114	115	116	117	118	119	120
A.	B	A	A	C	C	A	D	D	D	A	B	D	A	A	C

Q.	121	122	123	124	125	126	127	128	129	130	131	132	133	134	135
A.	D	D	B	C	A	B	C	C	A	C	D	C	A	A	D

Q.	136	137	138	139	140	141	142	143	144	145	146	147	148	149	150
A.	D	D	D	A	B	D	B	C	A	C	C	D	A	D	B

Answers and Explanations

1. D - The P wave on an EKG represents atrial depolarization.

2. D - A positive Trousseau's sign indicates hypocalcemia and is elicited by tetany in the arm when an inflated blood pressure cuff is applied to the arm for three minutes.

3. A - The addition of blue dye to formula to detect for aspiration is *no longer* considered a safe, standard practice. Several potential deaths may have been associated with the systemic absorption of blue dye in patients who were acutely ill or septic.

4. D - The secretory phase of the menstrual cycle begins with ovulation and occurs on days 15 to 26 of the woman's cycle. As the corpus luteum is formed, it secretes progesterone and some estrogen, causing the endometrial glands to produce nourishing fluid in preparation for a fertilized ovum. If fertilization does not occur, the ischemic phase begins (days 26 to 28).

5. D - Hodgkin's and non-Hodgkin's lymphomas are malignancies that involve lymph tissues. Multiple myeloma occurs because of a malignancy in plasma cells. The malignant plasma cells occupy more and more space, leading the the destruction of bone marrow. Multiple myeloma's effect is indirect, it is the only condition that describes a malignancy of plasma cells.

6. A - The patient with a cast that feels tight is at risk for circulation impairment and peripheral nerve damage. The needs of patients who have pain or are awaiting discharge are important, and the nurse will want to address these as soon as possible, but these concerns are less urgent than the potential risks to the patient with the tight cast.

7. A - Hypotension, not hypertension, is a clinical manifestation of this condition due to a decrease in venous return, and hyper-resonance, not hypo-resonance, occurs over pneumothorax.

8.   C - Ventricular tachycardia and ventricular fibrillation can both be corrected by defibrillation. Defibrillation coordinates electrical activity in the heart by suddenly shocking and overriding all other electrical signals, allowing the heart's conductive system to be coordinated electrical activity.

9.   C - Hemoglobin A1C is an indicator of blood glucose control during the previous three months. Recommended glycemic target goals for adults with diabetes include an A1C of less than 7.0%, preprandial (before meals) glucose levels of 70-130 mg/dL, and postprandial (after meals) glucose levels of less than 180 mg/dL.

10.   C - Albumin is a protein made by the liver that keeps fluid from leaking out of blood vessels, nourishes tissues, and transports hormones, vitamins, drugs, and substances like calcium throughout the body.

11.   B - Frequent dressing changes around the Penrose drain are required to protect the skin against breakdown from the urinary drainage. If urinary drainage is excessive, an ostomy pouch may be placed over the drain to protect the skin.

12.   D - Autoimmune disorders most often start in a system other than the immune system, but the immune system is involved because of the body's normal response to a threat. The immune system starts to attack the body's own cells.

13.   C - Phenytoin is a sodium channel blocker used in the prevention of seizure activity; it stabilizes neuronal membranes. Levels must be closely monitored in patients taking this drug; therapeutic level is within 10-20 mcg/mL.

14.   A - The purified protein derivative (PPD) intradermal skin test does not differentiate between active and dormant infections. If a positive reaction occurs, a sputum smear and culture, as well as a chest X-ray, are necessary to provide more information. Although the area of redness is measured in 3 days (48-72 hours after injection), a second test may be needed; neither test indicates that tuberculosis (TB) is active.

15.   C - Acute coronary syndrome is a term used to describe an array of myocardial ischemic conditions associated with sudden, reduced blood flow to the heart. It is primarily caused by *thrombus formation in narrowed coronary arteries*.

16.   C - Ketones are a chemical produced when the body breaks down body fat for energy. This can occur when there is no insulin to transport sugar into the cells for them to use for energy. Ketones in the urine is a sign that the body is using fat for energy instead of using glucose because not enough insulin is available to use glucose for energy. The presence of ketones in the urine is much more common in type 1 diabetes mellitus (DM) when insulin is not produced than in type 2 DM where insulin production is only reduced or where sensitivity to insulin is decreased.

17.   A - The liver is the largest internal organ, located in the right upper quadrant (the skin is the largest organ, but is external).

18.   D - An active outbreak of genital herpes simplex in the mother is potentially fatal to an infant; infection may be contracted during vaginal delivery, and therefore C-section is indicated with active herpes outbreaks.

19.   B - Diphenhydramine hydrochloride (Benadryl) reaches its peak effect 1-4 hours after administration. This medication is an antihistamine and works by blocking histamine release. It is used for symptomatic relief of various allergic symptoms and as an adjunct to epinephrine in anaphylaxis.

20.   C - Deep tendon reflex testing is part of the neurological assessment of a patient; reflexes are involuntary motor responses by the nervous system to a specific stimulus. Responses are graded on a 0 to 4+ scale. Grade 1+: hypoactive

21.   A - A hemothorax is a collection of blood in the pleural space (from blunt or penetrating trauma).

22. B - Brain natriuretic peptide (BNP) is an endogenous chemical secreted by the ventricles of the heart in response to elevated pulmonary capillary wedge pressure, or excessive stretching of the heart muscle cells.

23. D - Type 2 diabetes mellitus (DM) is increasing exponentially, especially among the minority populations of the United States. Approximately 90% of the DM population is diagnosed with type 2 diabetes.

24. D - Liver damage in cirrhosis results in blockage of blood flow in the portal vein, and portal hypertension results. As a result, collateral circulation develops, and visible abdominal veins, hemorrhoids, splenomegaly, and esophageal varices are found.

25. C - Surgical interventions for BPH involve an experience of pain for the patient, which can come in varying degrees. Telling the patient that he will be pain-free after surgery is giving him false reassurance and inappropriate information.

26. C - Immunoglobulin G (IgG) is the primary immunoglobulin in human blood and makes up a total of 75% of all the immunoglobulins.

27. D - Chronic hypertension, not chronic hypotension, is a potential risk factor for a hemorrhagic stroke.

28. A - A CPM device may be ordered following a total knee arthroplasty (TKA) to decrease the risk of postoperative stiffness and improve knee range of motion (ROM). To achieve maximum benefit, the machine should be used at least 6-8 hours daily.

29. A - A non-rebreather delivers oxygen at a concentration of close to 100%. If the patient's O2 sat is still below 95%, then more advanced respiratory treatments are necessary, such as the application of positive airway pressure via CPAP or BiPAP. Intubation will also allow for application of positive airway pressure.

30. D - During assessment, the nurse will listen for bruits over the major

arteries (abdominal aorta, carotid, and femoral), asking the patient to hold his breath while listening for a bruit. A bruit is an abnormal buzzing or humming sound caused by narrowing or bulging vessels.

31. A - Antidiuretic hormone is an example of a neuroendocrine hormone; it has components of both the endocrine and the nervous system. It is synthesized in the hypothalamus and travels along axons that terminate adjacent to capillaries in the posterior pituitary.

32. C - Drainage from a stoma can quickly irritate the surrounding tissue (peristomal skin). Therefore, a solid skin barrier, with a pectin base or karaya wafer that has a measurable thickness and hydrocolloid adhesive properties, should be applied.

33. D - Serum creatinine measures the end product of muscle metabolism. There is little daily variation because of the relationship to muscle mass. Limited increases can be seen in persons with muscle wasting. Decreased GFR results in *decreased* filtering of creatinine and *increased* creatinine levels in the bloodstream.

34. D - A healthcare associated infection is one that is caused by exposure to an organism in a healthcare setting. Catheters are a common source of HAIs, and the patient who has the catheter comes from a healthcare facility. Additionally, change in mental status is a common symptom of urinary tract infections in the elderly.

35. C - Pronation is turning downward. Turning a part away from midline is external rotation. Turning a part toward midline is internal rotation.

36. D - While emphysema puts someone with COVID-19 at greater risk of respiratory complications, emphysema is not known to be caused by COVID-19.

37. B - While the patient's symptomatology may seem to also match left heart failure, the history of rheumatic fever makes aortic valve stenosis more likely.

38. C - The presentation of hyperosmolar hyperglycemic syndrome (HHS) is more prolonged and insidious in presentation than diabetic ketoacidosis.

39. B - An oral cholecystogram (or gallbladder series) is an X-ray examination to visualize the gallbladder. This test determines the gallbladder's ability to concentrate and store dye, and the patency of the biliary duct system. The patient may be asked to drink milk or cream to check for gallbladder emptying.

40. D - The *primary* function of the kidneys is to maintain a stable internal environment for optimal cell and tissue metabolism.

41. B - The patient is having shortness of breath that may be due to the transfusion. If the patient may be having a transfusion reaction, stopping the transfusion should be the first priority.

42. C - The purpose of the teaching is to help the patient prevent falls. Use of mobility aids and assistive devices, such as a hip protector, can prevent hip fractures if the patient falls. Throw rugs and obstacles in the home increase the risk for falls and need to be eliminated from the environment as much as possible. Exercise helps to strengthen muscles and improve coordination, but patients who are tired from too much exercise are also more likely to fall; therefore it is important the patient understands rest is important when they are feeling fatigued.

43. A - Chronic obstructive pulmonary disorder (COPD), not lung cancer, is the most common respiratory complication caused by smoking.

44. B - While aging is not in someone's control, advanced age is still a risk factor for coronary artery disease. Sedentary lifestyle, smoking, and hypertension are all risk factors of coronary artery disease.

45. A - Pheochromocytomas are rare tumors of the chromaffin tissue within the adrenal medulla that produce excess quantities of catecholamines.

46. A - A closed liver biopsy is an invasive procedure in which a needle is inserted through a *small,* not a large, incision between the 6th-7th, or 8th-9th intercostal spaces on the right side, and a specimen obtained.

47. B - A condom catheter is a non-invasive catheter that is applied to the external part of the penis and directs urine into a collection tube. Male patients who are alert and oriented without any contraindications are ideal candidates for condom catheters. The patient who has stress incontinence and is scheduled for an IV pyelogram does not have any contraindications and is a good candidate for a condom catheter.

48. C - Anemia is defined as a decreased number of erythrocytes (red blood cells), malfunctioning red blood cells, or both, with subsequent insufficient hemoglobin to maintain oxygen supply to the tissues.

49. C - Clonazepam is not a sodium channel blocker. It is a benzodiazepine, specifically a GABA receptor agonist, which increases inhibitory neurotransmitters in the prevention of seizure activity. It is the first-line drug for treatment and prevention of myoclonic seizures.

50. B - Adenocarcinomas account for up to 40% of all lung cancers. Lung adenocarcinomas usually begin in tissues that lie near the outer parts of the lungs (periphery of the bronchi) and may be present for a long time before they cause symptoms and are diagnosed.

51. B - An S3 can be a normal finding in children, pregnant females, and well-trained athletes.

52. A - Obesity reduces insulin binding at the receptor sites (insulin resistance), which leads to pancreatic hypersecretion of insulin and eventual pancreatic cell exhaustion.

53. A - Elevated ammonia levels caused by liver failure are the source of confusion or changes in mental status that occur with liver failure.

54. B - Trichomoniasis vaginitis is a persistent, protozoan sexually transmitted infection that is common in young, sexually active women.

55. A - Acute lymphoblastic leukemia (ALL) primarily affects children age five or younger, with most cases being in children ten or younger. On an adult floor, this form of leukemia would be the least likely to be encountered. AML, CLL, and CML all primarily affect adults.

56. A - Guillain-Barré Syndrome can be fatal, but most people do survive.

57. C - The patient with emphysema is usually anxious due to dyspnea related to mild hypoxemia and leans forward to facilitate breathing with the use of accessory muscles. Very little sputum is produced in emphysema, and the patient appears thin due to difficulty eating and breathing at the same time. Enlarged alveoli lead to the classic "barrel chest" deformity.

58. A - Norepinephrine is a vasoconstrictor and will raise the patient's blood pressure further.

59. C - Urinary potassium concentration is a diagnostic test for primary hyperaldosteronism.

60. D - An *increased* (not decreased) production of hydrochloric acid in the stomach, possibly due to an increased number of parietal cells (cells that line the inside of the stomach and produce hydrochloric acid in response to histamine, acetylcholine, and gastrin), can lead to the formation of peptic ulcer disease (PUD).

61. D - Erythropoietin is a renal hormone that stimulates bone marrow production of RBCs.

62. A - Systemic lupus erythematosus (SLE) is a systemic autoimmune disorder. Joint pain is often one of the first signs of SLE and occurs early in the disease process.

63. B - The medulla is the most inferior part of the brainstem. It is a continuation of the spinal cord in the brain and participates in the control of respiratory, cardiac, and gastrointestinal function.

64. C - Asthma causes wheezing in the bronchovesicular areas that is primarily present on expiration. This is due to constriction or edema in the small airways.

65. C - Stroke volume refers to the amount of blood that is ejected by the ventricle during one heartbeat.

66. B - Diabetic neuropathy causes nerve damage that reduces sensations, particularly in the lower extremities. This makes injuries go undetected for longer, which increases the risk of amputation.

67. D - Proton pump inhibitors, such as Prilosec, Prevacid, Aciphex, Protonix, and Nexium, work by preventing hydrogen ions from entering the stomach, thereby blocking all gastric acid secretion. They should be used as short-term therapies (4-8 weeks) in therapeutic doses as they can cause GI infections if used long-term.

68. A - The guidelines for initiating bladder retraining include assessing the patient's intake patterns, voiding patterns, and reasons for each accidental voiding.

69. C - Visitors who are feeling unwell should not expose the patient to their illness. Spending two minutes with the patient would potentially expose the patient; these visitors should not be allowed in the patient's room.

70. D - Osteoarthritis (OA) is the most common form of joint disease and a leading cause of progressive disability in older adults

71. C - Pulse oximetry evaluates the oxygen saturation of the blood by measuring the percentage of oxygen attached to hemoglobin. The result of a pulse oximetry reading can be altered by hypovolemia, cold appendage, faulty placement, patient movement, dark skin color, and acrylic nails

72. C - Asymptomatic bradycardia does not require immediate intervention, but does require monitoring, specifically cardiac monitoring.

73. A - Postprandial plasma glucose levels should be obtained 1-2 hours after the beginning of the meal. The recommended postprandial target goal for an adult with diabetes is less than 180 mg/dL.

74. A - The length of endoscopies varies, and it is also the least important educational tool for the patient.

75. D - If fertilization does not occur, the corpus luteum degenerates causing estrogen and progesterone levels to fall. Vasoconstriction of the spiral arteries occurs, the endometrium becomes pale, and the menstrual cycle begins again.

76. A - Human immunodeficiency virus (HIV) is a small particle of genetic material surrounded by a protein shell and is an RNA-containing virus.

77. A - In evaluating a patient with sudden onset of unilateral weakness, stroke should be suspected. A CT of the head will be necessary to evaluate if the stroke is hemorrhagic or ischemic, allowing for better understanding of how to treat the stroke.

78. C - A pneumothorax is an abnormal collection of air in the pleural space that causes an uncoupling of the lung from the chest wall; there are three types: tension, spontaneous, and traumatic. Tension pneumothorax is an accumulation of air in the pleural space under pressure, compressing the lungs and decreasing venous return to the heart.

79. A - To provide pumping strength, the wall of the left ventricle (left lower chamber of the heart) is considerably thicker

80. B - The only insulin that is able to be given intravenously is regular insulin. All other insulins must be given subcutaneously.

81. B - A gastrointestinal hemorrhage is defined as acute blood loss from the upper GI tract. "Acute" or "massive" bleeding is considered a loss of 25% of circulating volume (which is about 1500 mL in adults).

82. D - Peritoneal dialysis does require a dialysis catheter that is placed into the peritoneal cavity.

83. B - A macule is a flat, circumscribed area with a change in the skin color; freckles and measles are examples.

84. A - A limb encased in a cast is at risk for nerve damage and diminished circulation from increased pressure caused by edema or compartment syndrome. Signs of increased pressure from the cast include numbness, tingling, and increased pain.

85. B - The pharyngeal tonsils and the adenoids (lymph tissue) are located on the posterior wall of the nasopharynx and guard against invasion by organisms.

86. D - Hypokalemia (low potassium) can lead to adverse cardiac rhythms. A run of ventricular tachycardia (V-tach) that resolved by itself could be an indicator that the patient may go into V-tach (a potentially lethal rhythm). This patient should be assessed first, even though he is not currently in V-tach.

87. C - Diets which severely limit carbohydrates are *not* recommended in the management of diabetes mellitus. Percentage of calories varies and depends on individual eating habits, blood glucose, and lipid goals.

88. B - Psyllium is a bulk-forming agent and promotes peristalsis by increasing the bulk of stools.

89. A - Following a TURP, the patient should still be able to have intercourse. There is a small risk of impotence, but this is not something that is expected.

90. B - Hodgkin's lymphoma is considered to be among the most treatable of adult cancers.

91. C - Compartment syndrome can occur within 6 to 8 hours after joint replacement surgery, or it may take up to two days to manifest. It oc-

curs due to high pressure in a closed fascial space due to swelling, and the result is decreased circulation.

92. B - Sputum produced by patients infected with Pseudomonas organisms is commonly bluish-green in color with a musty odor.

93. C - All of these patient complaints are serious, but when prioritizing, airway comes first, followed by breathing, then circulation. The patient who is struggling to breathe should be seen first, as all three of the other patients have complaints related to circulation.

94. A - Adrenocortical hypofunction results in decreased, or absent production of adrenocortical hormones and is known as Addison's Disease; this condition involves the destruction of the adrenal cortex and is autoimmune in nature, typically resulting from an infection (TB, CMV, fungi), HIV, hemorrhage, or infiltrative disorders.

95. D - Nuclear imaging scans show the size, shape, and position of organs. They may also identify functional disorders and structural defects; gastric emptying studies and liver/spleen scans are examples.

96. B - Pre-renal causes of AKI are causes that do not occur in the kidneys, and occur due to factors that occur before blood begins to be filtered by the kidneys. Hemorrhagic shock is a pre-renal cause of AKI, and causes decreased blood flow to the kidneys.

97. D - Petechiae presents as a rash that consists of tiny, pinpoint, flat red spots and can indicate bleeding in the capillary beds.

98. C - "RICE" stands for Rest, Ice, Compress, Elevate. Musculoskeletal injuries, such as sprains and strains, require immediate, appropriate treatment (RICE) during the first 72 hours to help ensure an optimal outcome.

99. B - A pulmonary embolism is an obstruction of the pulmonary vascular bed by a dislodged venous thrombus. The patient may experience tachypnea and tachycardia, syncope and cyanosis, crackles upon

lung auscultation, dyspnea, coughing up blood or pink, frothy sputum, pleuritic chest pain, anxiety and a sense of doom, hemoptysis, and low-grade fever.

100. C - An MI occurs when there is an abrupt loss of blood flow to the myocardial muscle, resulting in ischemia and eventual tissue necrosis. The most critical period after MI is within the first *6 to 24 hours* due to cardiac arrhythmias.

101. B - Exophthalmos, or protrusion of the eyes, is commonly seen with Grave's disease due to fatty build up behind the eyes.

102. B - Hepatitis is an inflammation of the liver, usually caused by one of six viruses (A, B, C, D, E, and G), or can be drug or alcohol induced. HVA is spread through the fecal/oral route. It is usually spread by water or food (especially seafood) contaminated by sewage (infected feces). Shellfish which have not been sufficiently cooked is a relatively common source. It may also be spread through close contact with an infectious person.

103. B - Kidney stones may cause trauma to the lining of the ureter that causes occult blood, which can be detected through urinalysis.

104. A - An allograft, sometimes referred to as a homograft, is skin of the same species donor.

105. D - Dual energy x-ray absorptiometry (DEXA) is the gold standard for diagnosis of osteoporosis.

106. B - Rhonchi are continuous low-pitched, rattling lung sounds that often resemble snoring. Obstruction or secretions in larger airways are frequent causes of rhonchi. They can be heard in patients with chronic obstructive pulmonary disease (COPD), bronchiectasis, pneumonia, chronic bronchitis, or cystic fibrosis.

107. A - Myoglobin is a small, oxygen-binding protein found in heart and

skeletal muscle. When heart or skeletal muscle is injured, myoglobin is released into the blood.

108. A - NPH is an intermediate-acting insulin, with an onset of 2 to 4 hours, and a peak of 6 to 10 hours; it can last up to 18 hours.

109. C - An ulcer in the stomach is known as a gastric ulcer while an ulcer that develops in the duodenum, the beginning of the small intestine, is known as a duodenal ulcer. Patients diagnosed with duodenal ulcers usually experience *no appetite changes, with minimal to no weight loss.*

110. C - Glomerulonephritis is a bilateral inflammation of the glomeruli within the kidneys and is typically caused by an immunologic reaction to an antigen. The sedimentation rate is *increased* due to inflammation.

111. A - Antibody tests are the most common method of diagnosing HIV. Diagnostic *confirmatory* tests include the western blot, which is the most common confirmatory test, and the indirect immunofluorescence assay.

112. D - Osteophytes (bone spurs) are extra pieces of bone that form as a result of insult or injury to the bone. Osteoblasts are the basic bone-forming cells. Osteoclasts participate in bone remodeling by breaking down bone tissue.

113. D - Tuberculosis (TB) is definitively diagnosed through culture and isolation of *Mycobacterium tuberculosis* (pulmonary organism causing TB).

114. D - Prinzmetal's angina is caused by spasms in the coronary arteries, not by arteriosclerosis. Angina is the clinical manifestation of reversible myocardial ischemia, which comes from either an increased demand for oxygen or decreased supply of oxygen.

115. A - Pheochromocytomas are typically individual, encapsulated tumors that are easily accessible surgically, making surgery on these tumors more likely to be successful than with many types of cancers.

116. B - Hemoglobin is a measure of the concentration of hemoglobin in plasma. During the initial phase of an acute bleed, hemoglobin will remain normal because, while the amount of blood and plasma is reduced, the concentration of hemoglobin is initially unchanged.

117. D - Polycystic kidney disease (PKD) is an inherited disorder characterized by multiple, bilateral, grape-like clusters of fluid-filled cysts that replace normal kidney tissue. These grape-like cysts contain serous fluid, blood, and urine.

118. A - The five layers of the epidermis from the innermost layer to the outermost layer are the:

   a. Stratum germinativum or stratum basale (innermost layer)
   b. Stratum spinosum
   c. Stratum granulosum
   d. Stratum lucidum (specific to the palms of the hands and soles of the feet)
   e. Stratum corneum (outermost layer).

119. A - MG is an acquired autoimmune disease characterized by weakness of skeletal muscles and fatigability that worsens with exercise and improves with rest. Ocular muscles are the most commonly affected muscle region, with ptosis, diplopia, ocular palsy, and nystagmus frequently manifested in patients with MG. Facial and respiratory muscle regions may also be involved.

120. C - Salmeterol is a long-acting beta-adrenergic agonist administered by inhalation and used for long-term control of bronchospasm; it should not be used for quick relief, rescue therapy.

121. D - Cardiomyopathy is commonly grouped into three categories: dilated, hypertrophic, and restrictive. Dilated cardiomyopathy is the most common type and involves enlargement of all cardiac chambers and systolic dysfunction.

122. D - Cushing's syndrome is the result of oversecretion of adrenocorti-

cal hormones. Cortisol is the primary glucocorticoid produced by the adrenal gland. Hyperglycemia (glucose intolerance), which develops from glucocorticoid excess, is a manifestation of Cushing's syndrome. With successful treatment of the disorder, serum glucose levels decline.

123. B - Chronic liver failure is defined as a progressive destruction of hepatic cells with replacement by nonfunctioning fibrotic tissue. Ascites (insufficient protein in capillaries causes plasma to seep into the abdominal cavity) develops with increasing loss of liver function. The enlarged abdomen can result in severe respiratory distress.

124. C - BUN measures urea, an end product of nitrogen metabolism. An elevated BUN is indicative of uremia, which is toxic to the CNS and causes mental cloudiness and confusion and can result in a loss of consciousness.

125. A - CML has a slow, insidious onset; the presence of the Philadelphia chromosome is definitive for diagnosing CML and is present in > 90% of patients, and over 50% of patients present with white blood cell counts > 100,000 uL. Symptoms may include marked lymphadenopathy, splenomegaly, and/or hepatomegaly; LUQ pain, abdominal fullness, fatigue, anorexia, and weight loss.

126. B - Plantarflexion is flexion of the ankle down toward the ground (pointed toes).

127. C - An PaO2 measures the amount of oxygen dissolved in the bloodstream. The patient's PaO2 should be between 80-100 mmHg. The PaO2 in an ABG does not require comparison with the pH to understand it further.

128. C - Upper back pain can be a presenting symptom of a myocardial infarction (MI). An immediate EKG will help to determine if an MI is causing the sudden pain.

129. A - The thyroid (not the parathyroid gland) consists of two lobes joined by a thin isthmus. The parathyroid gland consists of four small

glands located close to, or embedded in, the posterior portion of the thyroid and is responsible for secreting parathyroid hormone, which is essential for calcium regulation.

130. C - Esophageal obstruction is a blockage of the esophagus most commonly caused by GERD or, in rare cases, achalasia, which is a rare condition where esophageal peristalsis is absent with subsequent incomplete esophageal relaxation. Esophageal narrowing is normally asymptomatic until the narrowing is quite advanced. Painful swallowing is only noted as the disease progresses, along with the inability to belch.

131. D - Malignant ovarian tumors are linked to nulliparity, infertility, endometriosis, celibacy, use of talc on perineum, high-fat diet, family history, and previous breast or colon cancer

132. C - Plaque psoriasis appears as red, sharply defined plaques (primary lesions) covered with silvery scales (secondary lesions) predominately found on the scalp, elbows, knees, palms and soles, and nail.

133. A - Osteoarthritis (OA) is the most common form of articular (joint) disease and leading cause of progressive disability and pain in older adults.

134. A - Pneumonia that involves an entire lobe of the lung is classified as lobar pneumonia.

135. D - ACE inhibitors, such as captopril, can cause spontaneous angioedema, even after being taken safely for years. While the other options may cause angioedema as any medications could, ACE inhibitors are the most likely to cause this.

136. D - Hemoglobin A1C gives a general indication of an individual's blood glucose control over a 3 month period.

137. D - Appropriate management of symptoms improves nutritional status and quality of life. For diarrhea, well-cooked, easy-to-digest foods such as bananas, applesauce, rice, Jell-O, noodles, cooked carrots, and

canned peaches are suggested. Foods high in potassium should be encouraged, such as potatoes, bananas, fish, and meat.

138. D - Kidney stones can form from stasis of urine in the kidneys or ureters, but emptying your bladder frequently does not significantly reduce urinary stasis that is proximal to the bladder.

139. A - A rich source of iron is needed in the diet for a patient with iron-deficient anemia, and eggs are high in iron. Other foods high in iron include liver, shellfish, shrimp, and tuna.

140. B - Lordosis is posterior concavity of the lumbar spine (swayback).

141. D - The patient must be able to follow directions for pulmonary function testing to be completed. Some measurements are very dependent upon patient effort. If the patient is confused and unable to follow direction, the testing will need to be postponed.

142. B - A diagnosis of hypertension requires using the average of blood pressure readings from at least two separate occasions.

143. C - Syndrome of inappropriate antidiuretic hormone (SIADH) results from hypersecretion (*not* suppression) of antidiuretic hormone (ADH) and is characterized by hyponatremia (*not* hypernatremia) and increased urinary hyperosmolality caused by the sustained release of ADH in the absence of osmotic and nonosmotic stimuli. Water retention progresses to water intoxication.

144. A - You should assess the new admission with acute abdominal pain first because he just arrived on the floor and might be unstable.

145. C - TURP is the most widely used surgical procedure for BPH treatment. Because it requires no incision, TURP is especially suitable for men with relatively minor prostatic enlargements and for those who are poor surgical risks.

146. C - Suspected deep tissue injury is defined as purple or maroon local-

ized area of discolored intact skin or blood-filled blister due to damage of underlying soft tissue from pressure and/or shear.

147. D - A Colles' fracture occurs within the last inch of the distal radius; the distal fragment is displaced in a position of dorsal and medial deviation, producing pain in the wrist. A Colles' fracture would have no effect on a patient's leg length or position, nor cause pain in the rib area. Extreme pain in the ankle following an injury would likely indicate a Pott's fracture.

148. A - When administering respiratory medications, bronchodilators should be administered prior to administering steroids. This allows the airways to open and improves airflow into the lungs, allowing inhaled steroids to penetrate deeper into the lungs, allowing them to be more efficacious.

149. D - Levine's sign is a universal sign of coronary artery disease. It is characterized by the individual placing their tightly gripped fist over the sternum.

150. B - Brain tumors can affect the pituitary gland, the gland that secretes ADH. This can lead to diabetes insipidus if ADH secretion is suppressed.

Practice Test Two

1. All of the following are normal processes of aging except:

    A. Dental loss
    B. Reduced taste sensation
    C. A weakened gag reflex
    D. Altered rates of insulin release

2. The hormone that works with estrogen to prepare the endometrium for implantation of a fertilized egg is:

    A. Follicle-stimulating hormone (FSH)
    B. Progesterone
    C. Luteinizing hormone (LH)
    D. Prolactin (PRL)

3. You are instructing a patient with sickle cell disease about the precipitating factors related to sickle cell crisis. Which of the following, if identified by the patient as a precipitating factor, indicates the need for further instructions?

    A. Stress
    B. Fluid overload
    C. Infection
    D. Trauma

4. You are providing teaching about recognizing the symptoms of a brain attack to a patient who has recently been diagnosed with Afib. The patient asks what the acronym FAST stands for. Which of the following answers is correct?

    A. Face, Arms, Speech, Time
    B. Facial drooping, Arm drift, Somnolent behavior, Thrombolytic treatment
    C. Flaccidity, Aphasia, Somnolence, Thrombolytics
    D. Focus, Assess, Schedule, Treat

5. It is normal when auscultating the chest to hear:

   A. Crackles in the peripheral lung fields
   B. Bronchial breath sounds in the peripheral lung fields
   C. Vesicular breath sounds in the peripheral lung fields
   D. Bronchovesicular lung sounds in the peripheral lung fields

6. You are caring for a 68-year-old male on a medical surgical floor who has dilated cardiomyopathy. The patient's vital signs are:

   - Temp: 97.4
   - Respiratory Rate: 28
   - Blood Pressure: 58/30
   - Heart Rate: 128
   - O2 Sat: 92% on 2L

Which of the following interventions should be your priority?

   A. Obtain an order for an intra-aortic balloon pump
   B. Administer a bolus of 1L NS STAT
   C. Facilitate the patient's transfer to the ICU
   D. Verify that the blood pressure reading was accurate

7. In adult patients with diabetes mellitus, blood pressure should be measured at every routine visit to the physician. Target systolic blood pressure for the adult diabetic under the age of 70 is:

   A. 120 mm Hg
   B. 130 mm Hg
   C. 150 mm Hg
   D. 160 mm Hg

8. Colorectal cancer has been associated with all of the following except:

   A. Smoking
   B. High intake of saturated animal fats
   C. Multiple colonoscopies

D. Obesity

9. Urine estrogen levels are typically used to detect all of the following except:

A. Hyperadrenalism
B. Ectopic pregnancy
C. Intrauterine pregnancy
D. Ovarian pathology

10. You are caring for a patient who has been diagnosed with Christmas disease who asks you what causes this condition. Which of the following responses is best?

A. "This disease occurs because you have clotting throughout your body, which depletes clotting factors and makes bleeding more likely."
B. "This condition is another name for hemophilia B and occurs because your body does not make a certain clotting factor."
C. "This disease is a complication of infections that are most common in the winter months."
D. "This condition is caused by high sodium intake and is often worse when you eat salty foods like the foods people eat over the holidays."

11. Which of the following statements about contractures is true?

A. Contractures are reversible with physical therapy
B. Contractures result from a shortening of muscles and tendons
C. Contractures are caused by joint pain
D. Contractures are caused only by spasticity

12. You are providing teaching to a patient who asks you what causes asthma. Which of the following statements best describes the pathology of asthma?

A. "Asthma is caused by an inflammatory process that primarily affects the alveoli."
B. "Asthma is known to be an autoimmune condition that causes intermittent edema affecting the airways."

C. "Asthma is a type of chronic obstructive pulmonary disorder that can be fatal."

D. "Asthma is inflammation in the airways that often is triggered by an irritant."

13. While teaching your patient about coronary artery disease (CAD), you explain that the changes that occur in this condition involve:

A. Accumulation of lipid and fibrous tissue within the coronary arteries
B. Formation of fibrous tissue around coronary artery orifices
C. Chronic vasoconstriction of coronary arteries leading to permanent vasospasm
D. Diffuse involvement of plaque formation in coronary veins

14. Symptoms of hypercalcemia in primary hyperparathyroidism are likely to include all of the following except:

A. Nausea
B. Anorexia
C. Constipation
D. Oliguria

15. Sucralfate (Carafate) is commonly used in the treatment of duodenal ulcers and GERD. This medication:

A. Suppresses the secretion of gastric acid
B. Forms a protective barrier over the ulcer site
C. Inhibits the action of histamine
D. Neutralizes gastric acid

16. You are caring for a 42-year-old male who asks you about his risk for cancer. Which of the following statements is incorrect?

A. "You can reduce the risk of colon cancer by getting regular colonoscopies that can detect cancer early."
B. "Because you are male, you cannot get breast or cervical cancer."
C. "Even people who live healthy lifestyles may develop cancer."

D. "Smoking increases the risk of many types of cancers."

17.   When caring for a geriatric patient, all of the following nursing measures are appropriate for preventing pressure ulcers except:

A. Massage the patient's skin over bony prominences to increase blood flow
B. Inspect the skin at time of admission, then daily
C. Use the Braden Scale during assessment of patient
D. Use a barrier protection cream for skin at risk for becoming moist

18.   The nurse is caring for a patient with a neurological deficit involving the limbic system. Specific to this type of deficit, the nurse would document which of the following information related to the patient's behavior?

A. Cannot recall wife's name
B. Is disoriented to person, place, and time
C. Affect is flat, with periods of emotional lability
D. Demonstrates inability to add and subtract; does not know who President is

19.   The point where the mainstream bronchi, pulmonary blood vessels, nerves, and lymphatic vessels enter each lung is known as the:

A. Hilum region
B. Sternal border
C. Carina
D. Septum

20.   The heart has four chambers, right and left atria, and right and left ventricles. On the right side:

A. The aortic valve marks the entrance from the right ventricle to the aorta
B. The atrium communicates with the ventricle via the tricuspid valve
C. The mitral valve separates the atrium and the ventricle
D. The wall of the ventricle is much thicker than on the left side of the heart

21. In patients with diabetes mellitus who have normal renal function, protein intake should be:

    A. 50% or more of daily caloric intake
    B. 30%-35% of daily caloric intake
    C. 10%-20% of daily caloric intake
    D. 5%-10% of daily caloric intake

22. Which form of hepatitis is spread through close personal contact or via the parenteral route?

    A. Hepatitis B (HVB)
    B. Hepatitis C (HVC)
    C. Hepatitis E (HVE)
    D. Hepatitis A (HVA)

23. All of the following are pre-renal causes of acute renal failure (ARF) except:

    A. Hemorrhage
    B. Kidney stones
    C. Burns
    D. Dehydration

24. This type of immunity is produced by the immune response itself:

    A. Natural immunity
    B. Passive acquired immunity
    C. Active acquired immunity
    D. Autoimmunity

25. You are caring for a patient with a fractured femur who is in a traction splint. Upon assessment, you note the patient is restless and disoriented with severe hypoxemia. Auscultation of the lungs reveal crackles in the lung fields. What is the most probable cause of his symptoms?

    A. Venous thromboembolism
    B. Osteomyelitis

C. Fat embolism syndrome (FES)

D. Compartment syndrome

26. The maximal amount of air that can be expired by normal breathing after maximal inspiration is known as:

A. Functional residual volume (FRV)

B. Vital capacity (VC)

C. Forced vital capacity (FVC)

D. Tidal volume (TV)

27. Which term is used to describe the ability of the heart's pacemaker to spontaneously depolarize?

A. Automaticity

B. Rhythmicity

C. Conductivity

D. Contractility

28. In shock, the endocrine system triggers the adrenal response, which is characterized by the release of what hormone that causes the heart rate to increase, the bronchioles to relax, and the stimulation of gluco-neogenesis?

A. Aldosterone

B. Epinephrine

C. Glucocorticoids

D. Norepinephrine

29. *H. Pylori* is a bacterial infection that can cause inflammation of the stomach mucosa and lead to peptic ulcers. Which antibiotic is commonly used in conjunction with bismuth (Pepto-Bismol) and metronidazole (Flagyl) as part of "triple therapy" to eradicate *H. pylori*?

A. Levofloxacin (Levaquin)

B. Cephalexin (Keflex)

C. Clarithromycin (Biaxin)

D. Ceftriaxone (Rocephin)

30. You are caring for a patient with chronic pyelonephritis. Which of the following statements by the patient indicates there is a need for additional teaching?

A. "I might need dialysis eventually."
B. "This might be caused by frequent UTIs."
C. "This might eventually go away and I won't have kidney problems anymore."
D. "I might need to be on antibiotics for several weeks."

31. Which of the following diagnostic studies indicates red blood cell size, color, and/or weight?

A. Reticulocyte count
B. Erythrocyte sedimentation rate
C. Red blood cell indices
D. Hematocrit

32. Heberden's nodes are finger joint deformities associated with which of the following conditions?

A. Osteoporosis
B. Gout
C. Rheumatoid arthritis
D. Osteoarthritis

33. For a patient with chronic obstructive pulmonary disease, which of the following nursing interventions would help maintain a patent airway?

A. Enforcing strict bedrest
B. Administering prescribed sedatives regularly and in large amounts
C. Restricting fluid intake to 1,000 mL/day
D. Teaching the patient how to perform controlled coughing

34. You are performing a shift assessment on your 72-year old male patient. While listening to his heart, you hear a sound right before S1. What can this finding suggest to you?

    A. This is an atrial kick and helps the heart beat better
    B. This is an atrial gallop and can mean something is wrong
    C. This is a ventricular gallop and is heard in healthy patients
    D. Nothing. This is a normal finding in the older population.

35. Which of the following conditions is a contraindication for metformin (Glucophage)?

    A. Pancreatitis
    B. Diabetic ketoacidosis (DKA)
    C. Allergy to glipizide (Glucotrol)
    D. History of splenectomy

36. Your patient is complaining of pain upon readmission to the medical-surgical floor following Roux-en-Y Gastric Bypass surgery (RYGB). When addressing the patient's pain, your response is based on the fact that:

    A. Hypersomnia is common in unrelieved pain
    B. Physiological measures are the most sensitive in bariatric patients
    C. Pain increases the immune response
    D. Pain decreases gastrointestinal motility

37. A healthy adult bladder capacity is:

    A. 700-900 mL
    B. 100-300 mL
    C. 300-500 mL
    D. 500-700 mL

38. You are caring for a patient who complains of joint problems who is experiencing decreased range of motion, bilateral joint deformity that is symmetrical, and inflammation, warmth, and pain in the affected joints. The patient has no other symptoms. Which of the following conditions should be considered first?

    A. Bone neoplasms
    B. Systemic lupus erythematosus (SLE)
    C. Rheumatoid arthritis
    D. Osteoarthritis

39. What is the greatest risk to consider when administering a thrombolytic?

    A. Hemophilia
    B. Anaphylactic reaction
    C. Intracranial hemorrhage
    D. Gingival bleeding

40. Which of the following is the most definitive way to diagnose active pulmonary tuberculosis?

    A. QuantiFERON-TB Gold blood test
    B. Chest X-ray
    C. Purified protein derivative (PPD)
    D. Sputum culture

41. You are providing care to a patient who was admitted to the medical-surgical unit after experiencing a myocardial infarction (MI). Which of the following statements is true related to this patient?

    A. The patient may be treated with metoprolol (Lopressor, Toprol) due to its positive inotropic effect
    B. The patient's oxygen saturation should be maintained at 90% or above
    C. Renal insufficiency/failure is the leading cause of death in patients experiencing MI
    D. The patient is likely to be treated with morphine sulfate, as it is the

most common narcotic analgesic used to treat pain in MI/acute coronary syndrome

42. Which of the following is true about diabetic ketoacidosis (DKA)?

A. DKA is caused by excessively high blood glucose levels
B. DKA is treated by a combination of insulin and oral hypoglycemics
C. DKA never occurs in individuals with type two diabetes mellitus
D. A patient with type one diabetes mellitus will go into DKA if they use oral hypoglycemics instead of insulin

43. Which of the following statements made by a patient with hepatitis C indicates the need for further teaching?

A. "Hepatitis C has fecal-oral transmission."
B. "I am at higher risk now for hepatitis B."
C. "Hepatitis C can be fatal."
D. "My hepatitis C can be cured."

44. You are caring for a patient who has an indwelling urinary catheter. Which of the following interventions is least likely to help prevent infection?

A. Removal of the catheter
B. Flushing the catheter at least once every three days
C. Educating the patient about catheter care
D. Performing daily catheter care with soap and water

45. You are assessing a patient who has complaints of a lymph node abnormality. Which of the following findings is most concerning?

A. The lymph node is smooth
B. The lymph node is not movable
C. The lymph node is well marginated
D. The lymph node is painless

46.   The nurse is assessing muscle strength of a patient during a routine physical examination, in which a five-point scale is used. The nurse determines the patient has a grade 4 in his right arm. What does this indicate?

   A. The patient is able to move the limb against gravity with some resistance
   B. The patient's muscle strength is normal
   C. The patient is able to generate a visible muscle contraction but no limb movement
   D. The patient is able to move the limb against gravity but not against resistance

47.   You are caring for a patient who has a chest tube. Which of the following findings indicates the need for intervention?

   A. Tidaling in the water seal chamber
   B. Dependent loops in the drainage tubing
   C. Continuous bubbling of the water in the suction chamber
   D. The wall suction is set at a higher level than the amount of suction that was ordered

48.   When teaching your recently diagnosed heart failure patient about diet prior to hospital discharge, which of the following modifications are appropriate to discuss?

   A. Decrease sodium, decrease cholesterol, increase fluid intake
   B. Decrease sodium, decrease cholesterol, restrict fluid intake
   C. Increase sodium, decrease cholesterol, increase fluid intake
   D. Increase sodium, decrease cholesterol, restrict fluid intake

49.   Intermediate-acting insulins are effective for an approximate duration of:

   A. 14-18 hours
   B. 3-6 hours
   C. 6-10 hours
   D. 24-28 hours

50. You are caring for a patient who has been admitted to the hospital for diverticulitis. The doctor has put him on a special diet to avoid irritation of the gastrointestinal tract and to decrease fecal volume. Which of the following types of therapeutic diet is this?

    A. High-protein diet
    B. Low-residue diet
    C. Mechanical soft diet
    D. Full liquid diet

51. The inability to reach the toilet on time due to environmental barriers or disorientation to place is known as:

    A. Urge incontinence
    B. Functional incontinence
    C. Stress incontinence
    D. Overflow incontinence

52. All of the following pain management medications are likely to be ordered during the first 48-72 hours (acute phase) of burn care for a patient with deep partial thickness burns of the face and neck except:

    A. IV acetaminophen (Tylenol) with codeine
    B. IV hydromorphone (Dilaudid)
    C. IV lorazepam (Ativan)
    D. IV morphine

53. You are training a nursing student who asks you about Huntington's disease. Which of the following statements is not correct?

    A. "Chorea is common in those with Huntington's disease."
    B. "Huntington's disease is a genetic condition."
    C. "The changes caused by Huntington's disease can only be diagnosed on autopsy."
    D. "Huntington's disease will cause personality changes and memory loss."

54. Pneumonia-causing organisms which are opportunistic include:

    A. Cytomegalovirus, Pseudomonas aeruginosa, Klebsiella pneumonia
    B. Pneumocystis carinii, Mycobacterium tuberculosis, Cytomegalovirus
    C. Pneumocystis carinii, Haemophilus influenzae, Klebsiella pneumonia
    D. Streptococcus pneumonia, Mycobacterium tuberculosis, Mycoplasma pneumonia

55. If the SA node becomes damaged and nonfunctional, which of the following is the most likely to occur?

    A. The heart will stop
    B. Another part of the heart, possibly the AV node, will become the pacemaker
    C. The ventricles will contract, but the atria will stop
    D. The atria will keep contracting, but the ventricles will stop

56. A 14-year-old female who had a minor illness two weeks ago presents with "feeling bad," rapid breathing, and fruity smelling breath. Which of the follow labs is most important to obtain?

    A. Blood cultures
    B. Creatinine level
    C. Blood glucose level
    D. Urinalysis

57. Which of the following statements related to Crohn's disease and ulcerative colitis is false?

    A. Crohn's disease creates a nodular appearance of the GI mucosa, sometimes referred to as a cobblestone effect
    B. Bloody diarrhea is more prevalent in ulcerative colitis than in Crohn's disease
    C. Fatty stools (steatorrhea) are more prevalent in Crohn's disease than in ulcerative colitis
    D. Major symptoms of Crohn's disease are abdominal pain and weight loss

58. The nurse is assessing a male patient diagnosed with gonorrhea. Which symptom most likely prompted the patient to seek medical attention?

    A. Cauliflower-like warts on the penis
    B. Painful red papules on the shaft of the penis
    C. Foul-smelling discharge from the penis
    D. Rashes on the palms of the hands and soles of the feet

59. A patient with herpes zoster is newly admitted to the hospital. Based on your nursing knowledge of this disease, which statement is correct?

    A. If a person has not had chickenpox, they could contract herpes zoster
    B. Herpes zoster can appear in a healthy person at anytime
    C. Herpes zoster can only be diagnosed by skin stains
    D. The virus is located in the basement membrane zone of the skin

60. Which of the following interventions will help to enhance mobility and recovery in a patient who has just had a total hip arthroplasty?

    A. The patient will need continuous passive motion (CMP) to help maintain range of motion
    B. The patient should try to move the hip for as little as possible for the first 48 hours until the swelling at the surgical site has decreased
    C. The patient should exercise by moving the leg side to side as far as it will go each way
    D. The patient should begin ambulating as soon as possible once they return from the surgery

61. You are providing care to a patient with chronic obstructive pulmonary disease (COPD) and are aware that:

    A. Airway obstruction in COPD is typically more pronounced on inspiration
    B. The barrel chest deformity often seen in emphysema is caused by copious secretions that are difficult to clear from the airways
    C. With adequate treatment and patient compliance, COPD is fully reversible

D. Pulmonary function testing that measures expiratory airflow limitation is key to diagnosing this disease

62. Which of the following cardiovascular conditions is the most common type of heart disease?

   A. Hypertension
   B. Atrial fibrillation
   C. Cardiomyopathy
   D. Coronary artery disease

63. Symptoms of Grave's exophthalmos include all of the following except:

   A. Light sensitivity
   B. Dry, irritated eyes and puffy eyelids
   C. Cataracts
   D. Bulging eyeballs

64. You are caring for a patient who underwent a bariatric gastrectomy in which 80% of the patient's stomach was removed. You know you must observe for signs of pernicious anemia (vitamin B12 deficiency) because:

   A. Extrinsic factor is absorbed in the lower portion of the stomach
   B. Extrinsic factor is secreted by the stomach
   C. Decreased hydrochloric acid production inhibits vitamin B12 reabsorption
   D. Intrinsic factor is produced in the stomach

65. The nurse is caring for a patient with kidney stones. Of the following, which is the most important nursing action?

   A. Limit fluid intake at night
   B. Record the patient's blood pressure
   C. Administer pain medication every 4 hours
   D. Strain the urine at each voiding

66. A patient is diagnosed with late-stage human immunodeficiency virus (HIV), and the patient and family are extremely upset about the diagnosis. The priority psychosocial nursing intervention for the patient and family is to:

    A. Tell the patient and family that raw or improperly washed foods can produce microbes and increase risk of infection
    B. Tell the patient and family to stop smoking because it will predispose the patient to respiratory infections
    C. Encourage patient and family participation in care and discussion about feelings related to disease
    D. Advise the patient to avoid becoming pregnant because of the risk of transmission of the infection

67. Which of the following best describes crepitus?

    A. A joint that does move smoothly
    B. A type of breathing pattern that occurs immediately preceding death
    C. A crackling or grating sensation
    D. Air trapped under the skin

68. Which of the following statements is true related to the sinuses?

    A. They are fluid-filled cavities in the facial bones that open into turbinates
    B. They assist in the filtering of inspired air
    C. They assist in the sterilization of oxygen
    D. They provide resonance during speech

69. All of the following statements are true related to enoxaparin (Lovenox) except:

    A. Route of administration is per subcutaneous injection
    B. It will cause an elevated INR
    C. It is contraindicated in patients with leukemia and bleeding disorders
    D. It prevents conversion of fibrinogen to fibrin and prothrombin to thrombin

70. Which of the follow is not true about diabetic ketoacidosis (DKA)?

    A. DKA can be caused when insulin use is omitted or neglected
    B. DKA can be caused by an infection or illness in someone who has type one diabetes mellitus
    C. Only patients with type one diabetes mellitus can get DKA
    D. DKA is a medical emergency and will likely be fatal if not treated

71. The nurse suspects an acute gastrointestinal bleed in which of the following patients?

    A. A 20-year-old with nausea, epigastric pain, and bradycardia
    B. An arthritic elderly woman, with a pulse rate of 132 and hematemesis
    C. A 90-year-old confused male with a pulse rate of 90 and a blood pressure of 160/90
    D. A 30-year-old female smoker with a pulse rate of 58 and abdominal distension

72. A patient with chronic kidney disease asks the nurse, "Why do I need my kidneys? Can't I just live without them?" The nurse begins explaining the function of the kidneys to the patient. All of the following statements are correct related to the function of the kidneys except:

    A. They eliminate wastes
    B. They control fluid and electrolyte balance
    C. They maintain homeostasis of the blood
    D. They secrete vitamin D

73. Which of the following is not true of systemic lupus erythematosus (SLE)?

    A. Individuals with SLE almost always have a butterfly rash over the cheeks and bridge of their nose
    B. There is a high prevalence of SLE in individuals who are identical twins and whose twin has SLE
    C. SLE affects multiple organs and body systems at one time
    D. SLE affects women more often than men

74. All of the following statements related to the femur are true except:

    A. It is the largest bone in the body
    B. It is the longest bone in the body
    C. It is located in the lower leg
    D. It is the strongest bone in the body

75. When trauma results in a lung puncture, air is allowed to pass into the pleural space. As the pressure in the pleural space approaches atmospheric pressure, the lung:

    A. Fills with fluid
    B. Is no longer able to remain inflated
    C. Hyper-inflates
    D. Rapidly re-expands

76. The heart sound that is best heard in the left fifth intercostal space (ICS) along the midclavicular line, and whose soft *lub* sound indicates closure of the tricuspid and mitral (AV) valves is:

    A. S1
    B. S2
    C. S3
    D. S4

77. A male patient with a tentative diagnosis of hyperosmolar hyperglycemic syndrome (HHS) has a history of type 2 diabetes that is being controlled with the oral diabetic agent, tolazamide (Tolinase). Which of the following is the most important laboratory test for confirming HHS?

    A. Serum osmolality
    B. Arterial blood gas (ABG) values
    C. Serum potassium level
    D. Serum sodium level

78. You are performing an abdominal assessment on your patient. In which order do you proceed?

    A. Palpation, percussion, inspection, auscultation
    B. Percussion, palpation, auscultation, inspection
    C. Inspection, percussion, palpation, auscultation
    D. Inspection, auscultation, percussion, palpation

79. You are caring for a 21-year-old female college student who receives hemodialysis three times a week. She tells you that she may not have time for her dialysis treatments during finals week, and says that she may need to miss a few treatments. Which of the following responses is the best?

    A. "How can we schedule your treatments around your studies?"
    B. "It's okay if you miss a few treatments, just be sure to resume them as soon as finals week is over."
    C. "I will ask the doctor if you can skip some of your treatments."
    D. "Dialysis is a form of life support. If you miss your treatments, you will probably die."

80. A patient with a history of iron-deficiency anemia presents to the emergency room with glossitis. The nurse is aware this patient has:

    A. Red and inflamed conjunctiva
    B. Inflammation of the tongue
    C. Inflammation and burning of the lips
    D. Jaundiced skin

81. Which of the following describes Buck's traction?

    A. Manual traction applied to an arm to reduce shoulder subluxations
    B. A type of skeletal traction that is used on an arm
    C. A type of skeletal traction applied to a leg
    D. A type of skin traction applied to a leg

82. A nurse understands that treatment has been effective when a patient with pleural effusion that underwent a thoracentesis has:

    A. Increased respiratory rate
    B. O2 sat of 95%
    C. Reported 0/10 chest pain
    D. Absence of dyspnea

83. A patient who is scheduled for coronary angiography states, "I want to be asleep during my procedure. I can't stand any kind of pain." Of the following, the nurse's best response would be:

    A. "You have to stay awake, but the procedure is painless."
    B. "You will have to be awake during the procedure so you can control your breathing."
    C. "Don't worry. You will be given medicine to make you very sleepy, and you won't remember anything."
    D. "It sounds like you're feeling anxious. What has your doctor told you about your procedure?"

84. Pituitary Cushing's disease is usually caused by a small pituitary tumor (microadenoma) producing excessive:

    A. Adrenocorticotropic hormone (ACTH)
    B. Cortisol
    C. Growth hormone (GH)
    D. Corticotropin-releasing hormone (CRH)

85. Of the following, which serum liver enzyme laboratory value is abnormal?

    A. ALT: 30 U/L
    B. AST: 95 U/L
    C. ALT: 10 U/L
    D. AST: 40 U/L

86. Which of the following options is the best treatment to reverse the effects of polycystic kidney disease (PKD)?

    A. Furosemide (Lasix) 40 mg PO BID
    B. Broad spectrum antibiotic therapy while cysts are present
    C. Kidney transplant
    D. Surgical drainage and removal of cysts as they develop

87. A patient has been diagnosed with iron-deficiency anemia. Which of the following pharmacotherapeutics is the physician most likely to prescribe?

    A. Hydroxocobalamin (vitamin B12) subcutaneously
    B. Ferrous sulfate by mouth
    C. Hydroxocobalamin (vitamin B12) by mouth
    D. Folic acid

88. The most common cause of low back pain (LBP) is:

    A. Degenerative disc disease
    B. Mechanical strain of the paravertebral muscles
    C. A herniated intervertebral disc
    D. Spondylolysis

89. All of the following are risk factors for developing lung cancer except:

    A. History of seasonal allergies
    B. Exposure to coal products or radioactive substances such as uranium
    C. Smoking
    D. Exposure to radon or asbestos

90. The peripheral vascular system consists of a system of intertwining veins and arteries which carry blood to and from the heart and lungs and also involves the capillaries and lymph system. Within the peripheral vascular system, the amount of blood flow to each organ and various tissue is directly related to the degree of constriction in the:

    A. Venules

    B. Arterioles

    C. Aorta

    D. Capillaries

91. What is the treatment for hyperparathyroidism?

    A. Radioactive iodine (RAI) therapy

    B. Spironolactone treatment

    C. Thyroid hormone replacement therapy

    D. Surgical removal of the glands

92. Which of the following describes a Mallory-Weiss tear?

    A. A tear in the pyloric sphincter

    B. A tear in the esophagus

    C. A tear or perforation in the small intestines

    D. A tear or ulcer caused by shear forces in the oropharynx

93. A female patient has just been diagnosed with human papillomavirus (HPV). What information is appropriate to tell this patient?

    A. This condition puts her at higher risk for cervical cancer; she should have a Pap smear every 6 months

    B. The potential for transmission to her sexual partner(s) will be eliminated if condoms are used every time she engages in sexual intercourse

    C. HPV causes lesions called *condylomata acuminata* that cannot be transmitted during oral sex

    D. The most common treatment is metronidazole (Flagyl), which should eradicate the problem within 7 to 10 days

94. The physician has just ordered ferrous sulfate (iron) for a patient with iron-deficiency anemia. Which of the following instructions is appropriate for the nurse to give the patient related to this new order?

    A. Ferrous sulfate may be taken with juice

    B. If the medication causes stomach upset, take with milk or an antacid

C. Ferrous sulfate may decrease the amount of thyroid medication the patient needs to take

D. Ferrous sulfate often causes hard, clay-colored stools

95. Which of the following is recommended by the American College of Rheumatology as the initial drug of choice for osteoarthritis (OA) pain?

   A. Acetaminophen (Tylenol)
   B. Ibuprofen (Motrin, Advil)
   C. Celecoxib (Celebrex)
   D. Aspirin

96. You are caring for a patient who has been diagnosed with pulmonary fibrosis. Which of the following questions by the patient indicates that she understands her disease process?

   A. "When will my lungs begin to heal?"
   B. "What dietary changes do I need to make to improve my lungs?"
   C. "Will I be eligible for a lung transplant?"
   D. "Why do the cells in my lungs make too much mucus?"

97. You are providing teaching to a patient who is being treated for atrial fibrillation (A-fib). Which statement made by the patient indicates that they understand your teaching?

   A. My A-fib will improve if I eat more foods high in potassium
   B. I will have to take blood thinners to control my A-fib
   C. I may need an implanted device that will shock my heart when I go into A-fib
   D. My heart beat is regular now, but it might become irregular again

98. Medications associated with the development of hyperosmolar hyperglycemic syndrome (HHS) include all of the following except:

   A. Insulin
   B. Corticosteroids
   C. Potassium-wasting diuretics

D. Phenytoin (Dilantin)

99. Asterixis is most likely to be observed in a patient who is hospitalized for:

A. Chronic liver failure with encephalopathy
B. Scheduled removal of bilateral cataracts
C. An emergency C-section
D. Knee replacement surgery

100. Between ejaculations, sperm is primarily stored in the:

A. Ejaculatory ducts
B. Vas deferens
C. Testes
D. Epididymis

101. You are caring for 21-year-old male patient who has just been diagnosed with immune thrombocytopenia purpura (ITP). He is a college football player and is considering a career as a professional football player. The patient asks you "What impact will this diagnosis have on my football career?" Which of the following responses is best?

A. "Tell me more about how anxious you feel, considering that you might not be able to play football anymore."
B. "With this diagnosis, you should not play football or any kind of contact sport unless you are cleared to do so by your doctor."
C. "If your platelet levels are low, you will have to take extra precautions while playing football."
D. "As long as your platelets are above 50,000, you should be okay to continue playing."

102. You are caring for a patient who was admitted to the hospital for a closed head injury following a motor vehicle accident. Which of the following interventions should you implement to help minimize increased intracranial pressure (ICP)?

A. Maintain the head of the bed at less than 10 degrees

    B. Elevate the patient's legs

    C. Group all nursing activities and leave the patient undisturbed for 2 hours

    D. Maintain alignment of the head and neck

103. Regulatory centers in the brain respond to stimulation from sensory receptors. All of the following statements related to sensory receptors are true except:

    A. Chemoreceptors respond to changes in pH, PaO_2, and $PaCO_2$

    B. Stretch receptors prevent excessive distension of the lung

    C. As pH rises, a patient is triggered to breathe more rapidly

    D. When PCO_2 increases, a patient is triggered to breathe more rapidly

104. The amount of force the ventricle must exert to eject blood into the arterial system is known as:

    A. Systolic pressure

    B. Diastolic pressure

    C. Afterload

    D. Pulse pressure

105. You are caring for a patient with a diagnosis of syndrome of inappropriate antidiuretic hormone (SIADH). Which of the following nursing interventions is appropriate for this patient?

    A. Encouraging increased oral intake

    B. Restricting fluids

    C. Administering glucose-containing IV fluids as ordered

    D. Infusing IV fluids rapidly as ordered

106. Which of the following conditions is not a common cause of gastrointestinal bleeding?

    A. Esophageal tears

    B. Peptic ulcer disease

    C. Esophagotracheal fistula

D. Esophageal varices

107. Which of the following statements related to leiomyomas of the uterus is true?

   A. They are tumors that develop from smooth muscle cells in the myometrium
   B. The incidence of these tumors increases after menopause
   C. These tumors become malignant, and treatment often includes cryosurgery
   D. They are more common in Caucasian women than in women of other races

108. The adipose layer of the skin is found in:

   A. Both the dermis and the epidermis
   B. The epidermis
   C. The dermis
   D. The hypodermis

109. This condition, which most often occurs in the lower lumbar vertebrae, is defined as a defect or stress fracture in the pars interarticularis (arch between the superior and inferior articulating surfaces of vertebrae):

   A. Spinal stenosis
   B. Scoliosis
   C. Spondylolisthesis
   D. Spondylolysis

110. The most important section of the chest tube drainage system is the:

   A. Water seal chamber
   B. Heimlich valve
   C. Drainage collection chamber
   D. Suction chamber

111. Heart rate multiplied by stroke volume equals which of the following?

   A. Mean arterial pressure (MAP)
   B. Cardiac output
   C. Central venous pressure (CVP)
   D. Systemic vascular resistance (SVR)

112. Which nursing diagnosis takes highest priority for a female client with hyperthyroidism?

   A. Risk for imbalanced nutrition: More than body requirements related to thyroid hormone excess
   B. Imbalanced nutrition: Less than body requirements related to thyroid hormone excess
   C. Risk for impaired skin integrity related to edema, skin fragility, and poor wound healing
   D. Body image disturbance related to weight gain and edema

113. Your patient, Mrs. M., has Crohn's disease and just underwent a total proctocolectomy with a permanent ileostomy 12 hours ago. You are completing an assessment and should contact the physician immediately if Mrs. M. has which of the following findings?

   A. The stoma appears red and shiny
   B. There is 150 mL of dark green output from the stoma
   C. The stoma appears pale and dry
   D. There is 100 mL of serosanguinous drainage from the stoma

114. You are caring for a 68-year-old woman who was admitted to the hospital with complaints of painless vaginal bleeding. You should make certain the patient is tested for which of the following health problems?

   A. Ovarian cyst
   B. Uterine or cervical cancer
   C. Endometriosis
   D. Hormonal imbalances

115.   Which of the following is least likely to occur from a Roux-en-Y surgery?

   A. Pernicious anemia
   B. Anemia from blood loss
   C. Iron deficiency anemia
   D. Aplastic anemia

116.   A patient is diagnosed with osteoporosis. Which electrolytes are involved in the development of this disorder?

   A. Phosphorous and potassium
   B. Potassium and sodium
   C. Calcium and sodium
   D. Calcium and phosphorous

117.   All of the following statements are true related to pulmonary rehabilitation for the patient with chronic bronchitis except:

   A. It may help increase activity tolerance
   B. It may enhance the quality of the patient's life
   C. It may help lessen dyspnea
   D. It may help improve lung function

118.   Infective endocarditis occurs when infective agents in the bloodstream are carried through the system and are deposited where?

   A. In the bundle of His
   B. On valve leaflets
   C. On the walls of the major arteries
   D. On the Purkinje fibers

119.   You are caring for a patient who has pituitary Cushing's disease. Which of the following treatment options will be most effective in providing long-term relief of the patient's symptoms?

   A. 40 mg furosemide (Lasix) PO BID
   B. Adrenalectomy of only the affected side

C. 20 mg dexamethasone PO daily

D. Brain surgery

120. Which of the following best describes dumping syndrome?

A. Peristalsis in the large intestines becomes involuntary, leading to fecal incontinence

B. Excessive biliary fluid production that results in loose, green-tinged stools

C. More than four loose bowel movements in a one hour period or ten within a twelve hour period

D. Food empties from the stomach into the duodenum much faster than normal

121. You are caring for a 18-year-old female who is on peritoneal dialysis. She presents with abdominal pain, rigid abdominal muscles, and fever. Which of the following conditions should you assess for first?

A. Ectopic pregnancy

B. Peritonitis

C. Sepsis

D. Dialysis catheter displacement

122. Which of the following nursing assessment findings is not a symptom of polycythemia vera?

A. Headache

B. Dizziness

C. Excessive bleeding or bruising

D. Shortness of breath

123. Following cementless total hip arthroplasty (THA) of the right hip, early mobility restrictions for the patient are most likely to include:

A. Full weight bearing on the right lower extremity

B. Physical therapy that starts on postoperative day two

C. Weight bearing as tolerated on the right lower extremity

D. Non-weight bearing on the right lower extremity

124. The respiratory center is located in the:

    A. Medulla oblongata and midbrain
    B. Medulla oblongata and pons
    C. Pons and midbrain
    D. Medulla oblongata and thalamus

125. Noninvasive diagnostic studies of the cardiovascular system include:

    A. MRI, phonocardiogram, nuclear cardiology
    B. MRI, nuclear cardiology, echocardiogram
    C. Echocardiogram, nuclear cardiology, thallium imaging
    D. MRI, phonocardiogram, echocardiogram

126. Potential side effects of sulfonylureas include weight gain and hypoglycemia. Hyponatremia is also a common adverse reaction to which of the following first-generation sulfonylurea agents?

    A. Tolazamide (Tolinase)
    B. Chlorpropamide (Diabinese)
    C. Metformin (Glucophage)
    D. Tolbutamide (Orinase)

127. In enterally fed patients, common offenders in causing diarrhea include:

    A. Antibiotics, and infections such as *C. diff*
    B. Infections such as *C. diff*, and sucralfate (Carafate)
    C. Antibiotics, and aluminum-containing antacids
    D. Antibiotics and narcotics

128. Which of the following considerations related to breast cancer is not correct?

    A. Heavy alcohol use increases the risk of breast cancer
    B. There are genetic risks for the development of breast cancer

      C. Common metastatic sites of breast cancer include the pancreas, brain, and spleen

      D. Early detection and treatment significantly impacts the prognosis

129. You are performing a skin assessment on a new admission and notice a semisolid, encapsulated mass extending deep into the dermis. What would be the best word to use to describe this lesion in your documentation?

      A. Nodule
      B. Cyst
      C. Papule
      D. Comedo

130. You are caring for a patient who has a femur fracture in which the fracture line runs parallel to the bone's axis. Which of the following best describes this type of fracture?

      A. Transverse fracture
      B. Impacted fracture
      C. Linear fracture
      D. Hardware-related fracture

131. The morning weight for a patient with chronic obstructive pulmonary disease (COPD) indicates that the patient has gained 5 pounds in less than a week, even though his oral intake has been modest. The patient's weight gain may reflect which associated complication of COPD?

      A. Compensated acidosis
      B. Polycythemia
      C. Left ventricular failure
      D. Cor pulmonale

132. Which of the following is true for vital signs in the shock patient?

      A. The pulse will decrease, and the respirations will increase
      B. The pulse will increase, and the respirations will increase
      C. The pulse will decrease, and the respirations will decrease

D. The pulse will increase, and the respirations will decrease

133. Which of the following is true when administering rapid acting insulin?

    A. Rapid acting insulin should not be given until the patient's meal is available
    B. Rapid acting insulin has an onset of 30 minutes
    C. Rapid acting insulin can be replaced by oral hypoglycemics if the cost of the insulin makes it impossible for the patient to use
    D. A sliding-scale dose of rapid acting insulin should be given before meals and a larger dose should be given at bedtime

134. Your patient, Mr. C., is scheduled for a gastric emptying study. You instruct him that:

    A. A small tube (NG tube) may be inserted into his stomach so the contents can be aspirated
    B. He may be asked to drink orange juice during the study
    C. He will not be able to eat or drink for 8-12 hours prior to the test or during the test
    D. He may be asked to drink barium during the study

135. Which of the following is not a risk factor for urinary tract infection (UTI)?

    A. Enlarged prostate
    B. Pregnancy
    C. Diabetes mellitus
    D. Glomerulonephritis

136. You are caring for an 82-year-old male patient admitted the previous day with COPD exacerbation. Since admission, he has not eaten well and refuses to get out of bed because he can't "catch his breath." During your assessment, you notice a 2-cm red spot with localized warmth located over the sacrum that is blanchable. The doctor orders a hydrocolloid

dressing for the patient's sacral area. What is the rationale for using this type of dressing?

A. It provides an antibiotic sponge to decrease bacteria and help the healing process
B. It contains a solution to clean the wound environment
C. It can be changed several times without damaging the wound bed
D. It protects the wound and encourages a moist environment

137. The shaft of a long bone is known as the:

A. Diaphysis
B. Periosteum
C. Metaphysis
D. Epiphysis

138. You are teaching your patient with emphysema how to perform pursed-lip breathing. The patient asks you to explain the purpose of this breathing technique. Which of the following explanations should you provide to the patient?

A. It prolongs the inspiratory phase of respiration
B. It helps promotes an open airway
C. It decreases the use of accessory breathing muscles
D. It increases inspiratory muscle strength

139. While obtaining subjective assessment data from a patient with hypertension, you recognize that a modifiable risk factor for the development of this disease is:

A. Smoking
B. Consumption of a high-carbohydrate, high-calcium diet
C. Family history
D. Hyperlipidemia

140. Which of the following tasks should the medical surgical nurse perform first?

   A. Administer metformin (Glucophage) to a patient with type two diabetes who has an A1C of 8.3%
   B. Provide a snack to a patient who took their rapid acting insulin 20 minutes ago, but whose meal has not yet arrived
   C. Complete the preoperative checklist for a diabetic patient who is scheduled for a washout and debridement of a foot wound
   D. Perform the admission assessment for a patient who is being admitted for a diabetic foot ulcer

141. An esophageal obstruction is defined as any blockage of the esophageal lumen. What is the most common cause of this condition?

   A. Infection
   B. Achalasia
   C. Esophageal tumors
   D. Gastroesophageal reflux disease (GERD)

142. You are supervising a nursing student caring for a 34-year-old male who has been diagnosed with testicular cancer. Which of the following statements made by the student to the patient requires correcting?

   A. "Testicular cancer does not typically lead to erectile dysfunction."
   B. "It may be necessary to surgically remove your testicle."
   C. "Testicular cancer is not normally painful."
   D. "Testicular cancer has a low survival rate."

143. The median age of onset of acute lymphocytic leukemia (ALL) is:

   A. 4 years of age
   B. 15 years of age
   C. 60 years of age
   D. 50 years of age

144. Which of the following conditions is strongly associated with the HLA-B27 antigen?

    A. Spinal stenosis
    B. Ankylosing spondylitis
    C. Osteoarthritis (OA)
    D. Fibromyalgia syndrome

145. A patient with streptococcal pneumonia is admitted to the medical-surgical unit. The patient in the next room is being treated for mycoplasmal pneumonia. Despite the different causes of the various types of pneumonia, all of them share which feature?

    A. Inflamed lung tissue
    B. Abrupt onset
    C. Elevated white blood cell (WBC) count
    D. Responsiveness to penicillin

146. Which of the following statements by a student nurse indicates they understand monitoring a patient who has just undergone cardiac angioplasty?

    A. "One of the primary concerns will be ensuring there is no bleeding at the surgical site."
    B. "We will need to watch for infection at the donor site as well as the primary surgical site."
    C. "Her chest pain may continue to worsen over the next 48 hours before it begins to improve."
    D. "She does not need to be on a cardiac monitor now that her arteries are open."

147. The lowest fasting plasma glucose level suggestive of a diagnosis of diabetes mellitus (DM) in nonpregnant adults is:

    A. 127 mg/dL
    B. 112 mg/dL
    C. 180 mg/dL
    D. 90 mg/dL

148. A patient is admitted with bleeding esophageal varices, and a Sengstaken-Blakemore tube is inserted orally to control the bleeding. Important considerations in caring for this patient include:

    A. Avoiding ever releasing the pressure of the esophageal or gastric balloon
    B. Monitoring the patient for clotting of the stent
    C. Being prepared to cut and remove the tube if gastric balloon enters the esophagus, obstructing the airway
    D. Avoiding performing oral care until the tube is removed, as this may dislodge the balloon(s)

149. The most frequently reported sexually transmitted infection (STI) in the United States is:

    A. Gonorrhea
    B. Syphilis
    C. Human papillomavirus (HPV)
    D. Chlamydia

150. Which of the following clinical manifestations would the nurse most likely expect in a patient with a diagnosis of thrombocytopenia?

    A. Smooth tongue, joint swelling, tarry stools
    B. Pallor, pruritus, tachycardia
    C. Bone pain, cheilitis, shortness of breath
    D. Hematuria, epistaxis, ecchymoses

Answer Key

Q.	1	2	3	4	5	6	7	8	9	10	11	12	13	14	15
A.	A	B	B	A	C	C	B	C	C	B	B	D	A	D	B

Q.	16	17	18	19	20	21	22	23	24	25	26	27	28	29	30
A.	B	A	C	A	B	C	B	B	C	C	B	A	B	C	C

Q.	31	32	33	34	35	36	37	38	39	40	41	42	43	44	45
A.	C	D	D	B	B	D	C	C	C	D	D	D	B	B	D

Q.	46	47	48	49	50	51	52	53	54	55	56	57	58	59	60
A.	A	B	B	A	B	B	A	C	B	B	C	C	C	A	D

Q.	61	62	63	64	65	66	67	68	69	70	71	72	73	74	75
A.	D	D	C	D	D	C	C	D	B	C	B	D	A	C	B

Q.	76	77	78	79	80	81	82	83	84	85	86	87	88	89	90
A.	A	A	D	A	B	D	D	D	A	B	C	B	B	A	B

Q.	91	92	93	94	95	96	97	98	99	100	101	102	103	104	105
A.	D	B	A	A	A	C	D	A	A	D	B	D	C	C	B

Q.	106	107	108	109	110	111	112	113	114	115	116	117	118	119	120
A.	C	A	D	D	A	B	B	A	B	D	D	D	B	D	D

Q.	121	122	123	124	125	126	127	128	129	130	131	132	133	134	135
A.	B	C	D	B	D	B	A	C	B	C	D	B	A	B	D

Q.	136	137	138	139	140	141	142	143	144	145	146	147	148	149	150
A.	D	A	B	A	B	D	D	A	B	A	A	A	C	D	D

Answers and Explanations

1. A - Dental loss is *not* a normal part of the aging process, but rather, the result of poor dental hygiene.

2. B - Progesterone is secreted by the ovaries and prepares the endometrium for implantation and allows the uterus to maintain pregnancy.

3. B - The patient with sickle cell disease should avoid dehydration to minimize hyperviscosity and instructions should include fluid intake of 4 to 6 liters of water daily. Nursing interventions during a sickle cell crisis include oxygenation, fluid replacement, and pain management.

4. A - The acronym FAST focuses on three symptoms of a brain attack, these include facial drooping (Face), arm drift or weakness (Arm), and speech changes or slurring (Speech).

5. C - Vesicular breath sounds are low-pitched, soft, breezy sounds heard over the peripheral lung fields; inspiratory phase is generally longer and more audible than expiratory phase.

6. C - The patient's vital signs indicate that he may be developing cardiogenic shock due to his cardiomyopathy. Transferring the patient to the ICU as soon as possible will be necessary for him to obtain the advanced treatments needed.

7. B - In the diabetic adult under the age of 70, the recommended target systolic blood pressure is 130 mm Hg.

8. C - Multiple colonoscopies has not been shown to increase the risk of colorectal cancer and can aid in the diagnosis of this cancer.

9. C - Human chorionic gonadotropin (HCG) is detected in a urine pregnancy test to ascertain intrauterine pregnancy (normal pregnancy).

10. B - Christmas disease is another name for hemophilia B and is caused by the body not producing sufficient amounts of factor IX. This condi-

tion is named after Doctor Stephen Christmas, and the nomenclature has nothing to do with the holiday season. Systemic clotting leading to depletion of clotting factor is disseminated intravascular coagulation (DIC), not Christmas disease.

11. B - Contractures result from permanent shortening of muscle, tendon, or scar tissue that leads to decreased range of motion (ROM) of a joint.

12. D - Asthma is an inflammatory condition that affects the airways by causing edema associated with the inflammatory process. This inflammatory response is often triggered by an irritant.

13. A - CAD is characterized by an accumulation of plaque, cholesterol, and connective tissues on the intimal wall (not orifices) of the coronary arteries (not veins) that leads to partial or total blockage of the artery. It produces thickening and hardening within the coronary artery with lipid, free fatty acid, and platelet aggregation.

14. D - Symptoms of hypercalcemia may include Constipation, Anorexia, Nausea, Polyuria (not oliguria), and Depression

15. B - Sucralfate, often used as a pharmacologic therapy in the treatment of GERD and peptic ulcers, forms a protective barrier over the ulcer site of the gastric mucosa. It also promotes bicarbonate and prostaglandin secretion and suppresses the growth of *H. pylori*. This medication is not recommended in the case of acute GI hemorrhage as it may obscure visualization during endoscopy.

16. B - While males cannot get cervical cancer, they may still develop breast cancer. Breast cancer primarily affects females, but it can occur in males.

17. A - When caring for a geriatric patient at risk for pressure ulcers, the nurse should inspect the patient's skin upon admission, as well as daily, and should cleanse soiled skin, *avoid* massaging over bony prominences where ulcers are likely to develop (massage can cause tissue

damage under the skin), moisturize dry skin, use a barrier protection cream for skin at risk for becoming moist, and minimize skin exposure to urinary incontinence.

18.   C - The limbic system, located within the basal temporal lobe, is responsible for feelings (affect) and emotions and controls emotion-related behavior.

19.   A - The major bronchi, pulmonary arteries, pulmonary veins, and nerves are the structures which enter and exit the lungs in the hilum region. Hilar lymph nodes are also present in this region. Both the right and the left lung have a hilum region which lies roughly midway down the lungs, and slightly towards the back. They are similar in size, with the left hilum usually found higher than the right.

20.   B - On the *left side* of the heart, the mitral valve separates the ventricle and the atrium; the aortic valve marks the entrance from the *left* ventricle to the aorta. The wall of the *left ventricle* is considerably thicker than the wall of the right ventricle to provide pumping strength.

21.   C - In patients with diabetes mellitus, who have normal renal function, there is little evidence to suggest that usual protein intake (10-20% of daily caloric intake) should be modified. With evidence of neuropathy, it may be necessary to restrict protein to the adult.

22.   B - HVC (formally called NANB) is spread through close personal contact or via the parenteral route and has been documented as responsible for as much as 70% of post-infusion hepatitis and hepatitis in hemophiliacs.

23.   B - Acute renal failure (ARF) is defined as rapid deterioration in renal function and is characterized by retention of nitrogenous waste. Causes of decreased perfusion in ARF include pre-renal, intra-renal, and post-renal. Renal calculi (kidney stones) are a post-renal cause of ARF

24.   C - Acquired immunity is produced by the immune response itself; it

results from exposure to an antigen and subsequent development of antibodies.

25. C - FES is the presence of fat globules that deposit in the bloodstream and move into pulmonary circulation; it is a type of embolism that is often caused by physical trauma such as fracture of long bones.

26. B - Vital capacity (VC) is the greatest volume of air that can be expelled from the lungs after taking the deepest possible breath by normal breathing.

27. A - Cardiac properties influencing output are:

  • Automaticity: Pacemaker ability (the ability to spontaneously depolarize)
  • Conductivity: Each cell has the ability to conduct impulses to the next cell
  • Contractility: Ability to sustain contraction and empty (make each cell shorter or longer)
  • Excitability: Each cell has the ability to contract on its own, to send out impulses to other cells without it first being stimulated from another source
  • Rhythmicity: Ability to spontaneously depolarize at regular intervals

28. B - Epinephrine (also known as adrenaline) is a hormone and a neurotransmitter. When the body is in shock, the endocrine system sends out an adrenal response, triggering epinephrine (a hormone secreted by the medulla of the adrenal glands), as well as norepinephrine, aldosterone, and glucocorticoids.

29. C - The combination of medications that is used to eradicate *H. pylori*, known as "triple therapy" is bismuth, metronidazole (Flagyl), and another antibiotic that is either clarithromycin, amoxicillin, or tetracycline.

30. C - Chronic pyelonephritis is a gradual, progressive disease that causes

permanent scarring to the kidneys. Chronic pyelonephritis will not spontaneously resolve. Chronic pyelonephritis can be caused by frequent UTIs, prolonged antibiotic treatment may be necessary, and patients who have severe chronic pyelonephritis may eventually require dialysis.

31. C - Red blood cell indices indicate red cell size, or mean corpuscular volume (MCV); color (amount of hemoglobin, indicated by mean corpuscular hemoglobin concentration [MCHC]); and/or weight, which is mean cell hemoglobin (MCH). Clinically, the MCV and MCHC are significant in labeling the various anemias and may be part of a complete blood count (CBC).

32. D - Bony overgrowths on the finger joint closest to the fingernail (distal interphalangeal joints) are called Heberden's nodes and are commonly seen in osteoarthritis patients.

33. D - Controlled coughing helps maintain a patent airway by helping to mobilize and remove secretions.

34. B - Gallops may be heard when extra heart sounds (S3 and S4) are present. S3 is an additional sound heard after S1 and S2, and is called a ventricular gallop. S4, termed an atrial gallop, may be associated with pathologic conditions such as myocardial infarction or heart failure.

35. B - DKA is caused by metabolic changes that happen when glucose is not able to enter the cells. Administering metformin will reduce the levels of sugar in the blood, but will not help sugar get into the cells. Someone who is in DKA should never receive metformin, and should instead receive insulin, which will move sugar into the cells, reversing the ketotic metabolic process.

36. D The consequences of unrelieved pain in patients include prolonged stress response, decreased gastrointestinal motility, decreased immune response, delayed healing, increased risk for chronic pain, and increased heart rate, blood pressure, and oxygen demand.

37. C - The bladder is a muscular storage pouch in the lower pelvis. The normal adult bladder capacity is 300-500 mL. While the bladder may stretch to hold more than 500 mL, this is not its normal, healthy function.

38. C - Rheumatoid arthritis is an inflammatory joint condition that is caused by autoimmune dysfunction.

39. C - Intracranial hemorrhage is significant risk that can occur with the administration of thrombolytics.

40. D - Testing for the organism that causes tuberculosis (TB), *M. tuberculosis,* in the sputum is the best way to diagnose active TB. A chest X-ray will not provide a definitive diagnosis of tuberculosis, but will provide useful information. PPD and the QuantiFERON-TB Gold test will be used to diagnosis TB, but cannot be used to tell if the disease is latent or active.

41. D - Metoprolol is a negative, not a positive, inotropic drug. The patient's oxygen saturation should be maintained at *95%* or above. Although renal insufficiency/failure is a complication of myocardial infarction/acute coronary syndrome, *arrhythmias* are the leading cause of death in patients experiencing MI.

42. D - DKA is ultimately caused because sugar is not able to get into the cells, making cells change from their normal metabolic process of using glucose to an alternative, ketone generating, metabolic state called ketosis. This change makes the blood acidic, leading to a myriad of health problems.

43. B - Hepatitis C does not increase the risk of hepatitis B. Hepatitis C can be fatal if untreated, is transmitted by fecal-oral transmission, and can be cured.

44. B - Backflow in the catheter, which would occur with flushing of the catheter, should be avoided. A catheter should only be flushed when necessary and should not be performed routinely.

45. D - Painless lymph nodes are more consistent with a cancerous etiology than they are with inflammatory lymphadenopathy.

46. A - Muscle function testing provides information on strength and movement patterns. A five-point scale is traditionally used, in which a grade 5 muscle strength is normal. This patient is graded 4, meaning he can move against gravity with some resistance.

47. B - Dependent loops in the drainage tubing can allow fluid to accumulate in the tubing, affecting the function of the system.

48. B - The patient with heart failure retains sodium and water. Eating too much salt (sodium) causes the body to keep or retain too much water, worsening the fluid buildup that happens with heart failure. Therefore, the continued care and management of this patient needs to include a low sodium, fluid restricted diet.

49. A - Intermediate-acting insulin (i.e., NPH) has an onset of 2 to 4 hours with a peak of 6 to 10 hours, and a maximal duration of 14 to 18 hours.

50. B - The low-residue diet is used after acute phases of inflammatory bowel disease, regional enteritis, diverticulitis, and after some bowel surgeries. Foods included in a low-residue diet often include those which are allowed in a soft diet with the following modifications: limit milk/milk products to 2 cups daily; avoid most fruits and vegetables (fruit and vegetable juices are allowed); use only refined bread and cereal products (avoid whole grain products); avoid all seeds and nuts. If a patient is to be on a low-residue diet long-term, a multivitamin or liquid oral supplement is recommended.

51. B - There are five types of incontinence: functional, stress, urge, overflow, and mixed incontinence. *Functional incontinence is the inability to reach the toilet on time due to environmental barriers or disorientation to place.* These patients are potentially continent individuals who cannot or will not reach the toilet in time.

52.   A - Acetaminophen (Tylenol) with codeine and morphine sulfate (MS Contin) are usually administered PO (by mouth) to burn victims after the initial treatment or acute phase.

53.   C - Huntington's disease causes atrophy of the brain that can be seen on an MRI or CT. Alzheimer's disease can only be diagnosed on autopsy.

54.   B - Opportunistic organisms cause pneumonia in patients who are immunocompromised. They include, pneumocystis carinii, mycobacterium tuberculosis, cytomegalovirus (CMV), atypical mycobacteria, And Fungi.

55.   B - The SA node (referred to as the usual pacemaker), initiates atrial depolarization. If this component of the conduction system stops working, the atria and ventricles can continue to contract as long as the pacing is taken over by another pacer (likely the AV node).

56.   C - Rapid breathing, malaise, and acetone-smelling breath are all indicators of diabetes. Type one diabetes mellitus often occurs in juveniles after a minor illness. Testing the patient's blood glucose levels should be the priority. While the other labs may provide useful information, they will not help establish a diagnosis of diabetes.

57.   C - Inflammatory bowel disease (IBD) is a chronic inflammation of the GI tract and specifically refers to Crohn's disease and ulcerative colitis (UC). Steatorrhea is *more common in UC*, but it *may* also be present in Crohn's disease. Both conditions are associated with diarrhea, malnutrition due to loss of the absorptive surface of the gut, and abdominal pain.

58.   C - Symptoms of gonorrhea in men include heavy, foul-smelling, green-yellow purulent discharge from the penis, dysuria, and urinary frequency.

59.   A - Herpes zoster (shingles) is caused by the reactivation of varicella virus which has remained dormant in nerve root ganglion, not in

the basement membrane zone of the skin until reactivated. However, the herpes zoster virus *can* be spread from a person with the virus to someone who has never had chickenpox.

60.   D - Early mobilization of the joint is recommended to promote an earlier and more complete recovery.

61.   D - COPD is a disease characterized by airflow limitation that is not fully reversible; it is progressive and associated with an abnormal inflammatory response of the lungs to noxious particles or gases.

62.   D - Coronary artery disease (CAD) is a condition in which the arteries that supply blood to the heart harden and become narrow from the accumulation of plaque, cholesterol, and connective tissues inside the coronary vessels. This narrowing of the arteries (known as atherosclerosis) obstructs blood flow to the heart muscle and can cause a heart attack.

63.   C - Graves' exophthalmos is an inflammation of tissue (caused by a collection of mucoproteins) behind the eye causing the eyeballs to bulge. Exophthalmos may also cause pressure or pain in the eyes, light sensitivity, dry eyes and puffy eyelids, double vision, and trouble moving the eyes.

64.   D - Intrinsic factor, produced and secreted by the stomach, is required for the absorption of vitamin B12.

65.   D - Urine is strained to determine whether any of the stone debris has been passed. All debris should be sent to the lab for analysis to determine stone content and effective treatment course.

66.   C - The priority psychosocial nursing intervention for the patient and family is to encourage them to participate in care and to discuss their feelings about the disease with one another.

67.   C - Crepitus refers to a crackling or grating sensation that typical-

ly is noted with joints that do not move smoothly, sometimes called "creaky joints," or with air that is trapped under the skin.

68. D - The sinuses are air-filled (not fluid-filled) cavities in facial bones that open into turbinates. They do not assist in the filtering or the sterilization of inspired air; rather, they are lined with mucous membranes that assist in the movement of fluid and bacteria out of sinuses into the nasal cavity, as well as assisting in warming and humidifying inhaled air. They do provide resonance during speech.

69. B - Lovenox *does not* elevate the INR. Lovenox prevents the conversion of fibrinogen to fibrin and prothrombin to thrombin; contraindications include leukemia and bleeding disorders, and route of administration is per subcutaneous injection.

70. C - While patients with type one diabetes mellitus are more likely to get DKA, patients who have severe type two diabetes mellitus may also develop DKA. DKA is caused when a type one diabetic develops an illness or an infection or when insulin use is omitted or neglected. DKA is a medical emergency and can have a fatal outcome if not treated.

71. B - An elderly woman with tachycardia and bright red blood or coffee ground emesis is the most likely of these patients to have a gastrointestinal bleed. Since she is arthritic, she may also be taking medications that can cause gastric bleeding.

72. D - The kidneys are a part of the renal system and serve many purposes. They regulate the volume, electrolyte concentration, and acid-base balance of body fluids; detoxify the blood; eliminate wastes; regulate blood pressure, and conserve nutrients. In addition, they secrete renin and erythropoietin, which play a part in the function of the parathyroid hormones and vitamin D but do not directly secrete vitamin D. The kidneys also secrete potassium but work to stimulate aldosterone to stimulate the distal convoluted tubules to secrete serum potassium.

73.   A - SLE does cause a butterfly rash over the cheeks and the bridge of the nose, but this only occurs in less than 50% of patients who have SLE.

74.   C - The femur is located in the upper leg (the thigh); the lower leg is comprised of the tibia and fibula.

75.   B - The pleural space normally maintains a negative pressure, which causes lung expansion. When air enters the pleural space as a result of trauma, pressure in the pleural space approaches atmospheric pressure, and the lung is no longer able to remain inflated. As air accumulates in the pleural space, it compresses the lung, causing it to collapse.

76.   A - Heart sounds are the noises generated by the beating heart and the resultant flow of blood through it. Specifically, the sounds reflect the turbulence created when the heart valves snap shut. There are two normal heart sounds (in healthy adults) often described as a *lub* and a *dub*, that occur in sequence with each heartbeat. These include the first heart sound (S1 *lub*) and second heart sound (S2 *dub*), produced by the closing of the AV valves and semilunar (aortic and pulmonic) valves, respectively.

77.   A - Hyperosmolar hyperglycemic syndrome (HHS) is a serious metabolic derangement that often occurs in patients with diabetes (but can occur in those without any history of glucose intolerance) and can be a life-threatening emergency. It is characterized by hyperglycemia, hyperosmolarity, and dehydration without significant ketoacidosis.

78.   D - Always follow this order during assessment of a patient; begin with patient history, including pertinent past and present history of GI problems, current medications, and any previous surgeries.

79.   A - Hemodialysis is a form of life support, and the patient should not miss any treatments. Missing treatments can also lead to illness that can interfere with the patient's study and test performance. Asking the patient an open-ended question about how to best schedule treatments is the best response. The patient will also likely require teaching about the need to not miss dialysis treatments.

80. B - Glossitis is an inflammation or burning of the tongue; this symptom is specific to iron-deficiency anemia or vitamin B12 deficiency. Other symptoms include cheilitis, which is inflammation of the lips, headache, weakness, and paresthesias of the hands and feet.

81. D - Buck's traction is a skin traction that is applied to a leg, typically used to reduce discomfort caused by hip fractures or to immobilize a knee.

82. D - A pleural effusion is a collection of excess fluid in the pleural space, located between the visceral and parietal linings of the lungs; this condition occurs when the rate of fluid entering the pleural space from the visceral pleura exceeds the rate of removal by lymph vessels of parietal pleura.

83. D - It is most therapeutic to acknowledge the patient's feelings, find out what they have been told, and not to minimize fear. Sedation pre-procedure may be ordered. The patient should be taught about the use of local anesthesia for catheter insertion, hot flash as the dye is injected, and "fluttering" sensation as the catheter is passed.

84. A - Cushing's disease/syndrome is the result of oversecretion of adrenocortical hormones; it occurs when the pituitary gland makes too much ACTH. ACTH then signals the adrenal glands to produce too much cortisol.

85. B - Elevated liver enzymes may indicate inflammation or damage to cells in the liver. A normal AST level ranges from 7-40 U/L, and normal ALT levels are 5-36 U/L.

86. C - PKD is a progressive, genetic, incurable condition in which normal kidney tissues are replaced with cysts. The effects of PKD cannot be reversed, and kidney transplant is the only way to eliminate the effects of this disease.

87. B - Anemia occurs when there is insufficient hemoglobin to maintain adequate oxygen supply to the tissues. Iron is essential for the forma-

tion of hemoglobin. In iron-deficiency anemia, there is not enough iron available in the body. Ferrous sulfate is iron and is used as a supplement to treat iron deficiency anemia, typically prescribed in a pill form, orally, three times per day.

88. B - LBP is defined as pain in the lumbar region of the back. The most common cause of LBP is mechanical strain of the paravertebral muscles. The pain may be related to a single traumatic event but also may occur as a result of excessive micro-traumas. The other choices also cause LBP but are not as common.

89. A - Lung cancer is the most common cancer worldwide. Smokers are ten times more likely to develop lung cancer than non-smokers, and exposure to second-hand smoke, radon, asbestos, coal products or radioactive substances also put an individual at risk. Chronic lung conditions may pose an increased risk for lung cancer as well. Seasonal allergies do not increase a person's risk for lung cancer.

90. B - The arterioles have little elastic tissue. They contain smooth muscle tissue, which allows them to constrict or dilate easily. The amount of blood flow to each organ and various tissue is directly related to the degree of constriction in the arterioles.

91. D - When hyperparathyroidism (oversecretion of parathyroid hormone from one or more of the parathyroid glands) requires treatment, surgery is the treatment of choice and is considered curative in 95% of cases.

92. B - A Mallory-Weiss tear is a tear in the esophagus or in the esophagogastric junction. It is often caused by stress on the area, most commonly from excessive or strong vomiting. They are strongly correlated with alcohol or NSAID use.

93. A - HPV is the most common viral sexually transmitted infection (STI); (although chlamydia is the most frequently reported STI). Women with *condylomata acuminata* (HPV) are at risk for cancer of the cervix and vulva. Yearly Pap smears are crucial for early detection;

if diagnosed, Paps are necessary every 6 months to monitor for cervical changes.

94. A - Ferrous sulfate may be taken with juice, but not with milk or antacids because these reduce the bioavailability of the iron supplement.

95. A - Pharmacologic management of patients with OA includes analgesics, NSAIDs, and salicylates. Acetaminophen, however, is recommended as the initial drug of choice for OA pain, in doses up to 1,000 mg four times daily for persons with normal liver function.

96. C - Pulmonary fibrosis is a progressive disease for which there is no cure. The lungs will not begin to heal and dietary changes will not lead to improvements. Cystic fibrosis, not pulmonary fibrosis, causes the cells in the lungs to create too much mucus, leading to respiratory disease.

97. D - A-fib often returns after it has been successfully treated. A patient who had A-fib may develop A-fib again in the future.

98. A - Hyperosmolar hyperglycemic syndrome (HHS) is a serious metabolic derangement that occurs in patients with diabetes mellitus (DM) and can be a life-threatening emergency. Some medications associated with the development of HHS include corticosteroids, potassium-wasting diuretics (such as thiazides and furosemide), and phenytoin. Insulin is part of the treatment plan in the patient with HHS, along with fluid and electrolyte replacement therapy, and correction of the underlying condition.

99. A - Chronic liver failure is defined as a progressive destruction of hepatic cells with replacement by nonfunctioning fibrotic tissue. Encephalopathy represents end-stage chronic liver disease and is related to the accumulation of noxious substances in the circulatory system due to the inability of the liver to render them water-soluble for excretion in urine. Early manifestations of encephalopathy include subtle changes in personality, changes in handwriting, and *asterixis*, which is flapping tremors in the hands due to toxins at peripheral nerves.

100. D - The epididymis is a tube that connects the testicle to the vas deferens in the male reproductive system; it is a comma-shaped structure that curves over the testes and stores and carries sperm from the testes to the vas deferens.

101. B - Contact sports should be avoided for patients with ITP unless they are cleared by their doctor. The doctor will consider the patient's platelet count and risk of bleeding when making this decision, but in most situations will discourage involvement in contact sports.

102. D - Positioning the patient with increased ICP to maintain the head and neck alignment will facilitate cerebral spinal fluid drainage and prevent further increasing the patient's ICP due to impediment of spinal fluid drainage.

103. C As pH rises, due to decreased PCO2, the patient is triggered to breathe more *slowly*, not more rapidly.

104. C - Afterload is the end load against which the heart contracts to eject blood.

105. B - Syndrome of inappropriate antidiuretic hormone (SIADH) results from hypersecretion of antidiuretic hormone (ADH) from the posterior pituitary gland and is characterized by hyponatremia, in which the plasma sodium levels are lowered, and total body fluid is increased. Although the sodium level is low, SIADH is brought about by an excess of water, rather than a deficit of sodium. To reduce water retention in the patient with SIADH, the nurse should restrict fluids.

106. C - Esophagotracheal fistula is a lesion that allows for communication between the esophagus and trachea. While esophagotracheal fistulas may be associated with other conditions that make a GI bleed more likely, esophagotracheal fistulas themselves are not a common cause of GI bleeding.

107. A - Leiomyomas are also called myomas, fibromyomas, or fibroids; they are benign tumors that develop from smooth muscle cells in the

myometrium. Although they have an unknown etiology, their growth is related to estrogen.

108. D - The adipose layer of the skin is found in the hypodermis; it forms a subcutaneous layer below the dermis and contains a group of blood vessels; it attaches the dermis to the underlying structures and provides insulation, a reserve of energy, cushioning, and adds to the mobility of the skin over underlying organs.

109. D - Spondylolysis is a defect or break in the pars interarticularis (the arch between the superior and inferior articulating surfaces of vertebrae). It most often occurs at L4-L5 or L5-S1 vertebrae, causing pain in the lower lumbar area of the back.

110. A - The water seal chamber is the most important section in the chest tube drainage system because it prevents air from entering the chest cavity during inhalation and allows air to escape during expiration. It also assists in re-establishing and maintaining negative air pressure.

111. B - Cardiac output is the amount of blood pumped by each ventricle in 1 minute, calculated by multiplying the stroke volume by the heart rate. Normal cardiac output is 4-8 L/min.

112. B - In the patient with hyperthyroidism, excessive thyroid hormone production leads to hypermetabolism and increased nutrient metabolism. These conditions may result in a negative nitrogen balance, increased protein synthesis and breakdown, decreased glucose tolerance, and fat mobilization and depletion. This puts the patient at risk for marked nutrient and calorie deficiency, making Imbalanced nutrition: Less than body requirements the most important nursing diagnosis.

113. A - If there is an adequate blood supply to the stoma, the color is pink or red, and the stoma is moist, as a result of mucous production. The stoma will be edematous for the first 5-7 days postoperatively. A pale, dry stoma suggests ischemia of the stoma or bowel and must be reported immediately to the physician.

114. B - Painless, abnormal uterine bleeding is an early and common symptom of cancers of the uterus and cervix. Due to this finding, the patient should be tested for cancer.

115. D - Aplastic anemia is a type of anemia that occurs when red blood cells are not produced by bone marrow and is unlikely to be caused by a surgery affecting the stomach or intestines.

116. D - In osteoporosis, there is a severe reduction of bone mass; bones lose calcium and phosphate salts, becoming porous, brittle, and abnormally vulnerable to fracture.

117. D - Patients may benefit from pulmonary rehabilitation that includes a program of supervised, individualized, and progressive exercise. Benefits of pulmonary rehabilitation include better activity tolerance, less dyspnea, and enhanced quality of life.

118. B - Infective endocarditis (IE) is an infection of the endocardial tissue of the heart. The endocardium is the thin, smooth membrane that lines the inside of the chambers of the heart and forms the surface of the valves; therefore, IE affects the valves. IE occurs when blood flow turbulence within the heart allows the infective agent (organism) to infect previously damaged valves or other endothelial surfaces.

119. D - Pituitary Cushing's disease is usually caused by a pituitary tumor. These tumors are usually relatively easy to treat surgically, making brain surgery the treatment option that will most likely help the patient.

120. D - Food empties from the stomach into the duodenum much faster than normal. Dumping syndrome describes a condition where food empties from the stomach more rapidly than normal, leading to decreased absorption of nutrients and abdominal distention.

121. B - The patient's symptoms best match potential peritonitis, and the patient is at a high risk for this with a peritoneal dialysis catheter.

122. C - Polycythemia vera is an excess in red blood cells caused by a muta-

tion in a hematopoietic stem cell, and is characterized by a hematocrit of greater than 55%. Headache and dizziness are early symptoms.

123. D - Cementless prosthesis for THA are indicated for very active patients who place greater demand on the joint. Any limitation in weight-bearing is determined by the surgeon, based on the type of implant. Following cementless THA, the patient is most likely non-weight bearing (NWB) or toe-touch weight bearing (TTWB).

124. B - Respiration is regulated by the respiratory center (in the medulla oblongata and pons of the brain), and the autonomic nervous system. The autonomic nervous system regulates smooth muscles of the airways via the parasympathetic and sympathetic systems.

125. D - Noninvasive diagnostic studies of the cardiovascular system include MRI, phonocardiogram, echocardiogram, EKG, and chest x-ray.

126. B - Potential adverse reactions to chlorpropamide (Diabinese), a first-generation oral sulfonylurea agent, include increased risk of hypoglycemia, weight gain, hyponatremia, and disulfiram reaction.

127. A - In enterally fed patients, common offenders in causing diarrhea are more frequently associated with medications and other causes, rather than formula or feeding itself. Offensive medications include antibiotics, elixirs containing sorbitol, magnesium-containing antacids, phosphate and potassium supplements, lactulose, and any medications with a side effect of diarrhea.

128. C - While the brain is a common metastatic site of breast cancer, the pancreas and spleen are not. Early detection and treatment is very important for a patient with breast cancer and does impact the prognosis. Heavy alcohol use and certain genetic factors both increase the risk of breast cancer.

129. B - A cyst is a semisolid or fluid filled encapsulated mass that can extend deep into the dermis.

130. C - A linear fracture is a fracture in which the fracture line runs parallel to the axis of the bone.

131. D - Cor pulmonale, or right-sided heart failure, is a possible complication of COPD. Polycythemia and compensated acidosis do not cause weight gain. Left ventricular failure would be expected in pulmonary edema, not COPD.

132. B - In shock, the pulse increases (tachycardia) to help improve cardiac output, and respirations increase (tachypnea) to help maximize oxygenation of circulating blood.

133. A - Rapid acting insulin can cause hypoglycemia if the patient does not eat within 15-30 minutes. This form of insulin should not be given until food is available.

134. B - For gastric emptying studies, the patient is often asked to eat a cooked egg white or to drink orange juice.

135. D - Infection of the urinary tract is more likely in women who are pregnant or in men with an enlarged prostate. Diabetes mellitus increases the glucose content of the urine, making it more likely to grow bacteria and cause a UTI. Glomerulonephritis is inflammation of the glomeruli and does not cause UTIs.

136. D - Management of partial-thickness (superficial) ulcers such as the one described in this scenario involves covering with a noncontact layer, hydrocolloid hydrogel, or transparent film dressing as the wound tends to heal more quickly with a moisture-retentive dressing that is not changed as frequently as conventional dressings.

137. A - Long bones, found in the extremities, have many structural components. The diaphysis is the bone shaft.

138. B - In pursed-lip breathing (inhale through the nose with mouth closed, exhale slowly through pursed lips), the patient maintains open airways by extending the positive lung pressure during exhalation (not

inspiration), thus helping to prevent early airway collapse. Learning this technique helps the patient to control respiration during periods of excitement, anxiety, exercise, and respiratory distress.

139. A - Primary risk factors for hypertension include family history (non-modifiable), age, male younger than 55, female greater than 74 years of age, African-American ethnicity, high dietary sodium intake (not carbohydrates or calcium), diabetes mellitus, and smoking (modifiable)

140. B - Rapid acting insulin has an onset of 15 minutes and may peak at 30 minutes. A patient who has taken rapid acting insulin may become hypoglycemic without food and should be given a snack if their meal tray is delayed. While the other patients also require attention, the potential risk of hypoglycemia makes this patient a priority.

141. D - Esophageal obstruction is most commonly caused by GERD (gastroesophageal reflux disease), in which gastric contents obstruct the esophagus. In rare cases, it can be caused by achalasia, which is an uncommon condition in which esophageal peristalsis is absent with subsequent increased lower esophageal sphincter pressure and incomplete esophageal relaxation; the outcome is obstruction of the esophagus. Other causes include esophageal tumors/cancer, strictures, bacterial/viral infections, or congenital anomaly.

142. D - Testicular cancer has a high survival rate of about 95%.

143. A - The median age of onset of acute lymphocytic leukemia (ALL) is 4 years of age, although it is seen in adults as well.

144. B - Ankylosing spondylitis is a type of arthritis in which there is long-term inflammation of the joints of the spine; the sacroiliac joint (between the spine and the pelvis) is also often affected.

145. A - The common feature of all types of pneumonia is an inflammatory pulmonary response to the offending organism or agent.

146. A - Cardiac angioplasty involves using a balloon to open clogged coronary arteries. Angioplasty is done by accessing the radial or femoral artery, causing a risk of bleeding postoperatively. Ensuring that no bleeding is present at the surgical site is one of the primary concerns following a cardiac angioplasty.

147. A - Criteria for the diagnosis of diabetes mellitus in nonpregnant adults include the following:

    - Symptoms and random plasma glucose concentration of > 200 mg/dL, or
    - Fasting plasma glucose level > 126 mg/dL following an overnight fast of at least 8 hours, or
    - A1C $\geq$ 6.5%, or
    - 2-hour plasma glucose > 200 mg/dL during an oral glucose tolerance test

148. C - Balloon tamponade is a temporary measure used when endoscopic and pharmacologic therapy cannot control the bleeding. A multi-lumen Sengstaken-Blakemore tube is inserted nasally or orally. The gastric balloon is inflated first; if bleeding is still not controlled, then the esophageal balloon is also inflated. Heavy scissors should be kept at the patient's bedside to cut and remove the tube if the gastric balloon enters the esophagus and causes asphyxiation. Never deflate the gastric balloon alone.

149. D - The Centers for Disease Control (CDC) estimates there are about 20 million new infections in the United States each year, and half of all new STIs occur in young men and women. Chlamydia is the most frequently reported STI in the US, with infection rates having increased over the past 20 years.

150. D - Thrombocytopenia is a condition in which there is a decrease in the number of circulating platelets to less than 100,000 uL to 150,000 uL. The patient may be asymptomatic, but most patients present with bleeding from mucous membranes or skin. Manifestations may include:

- Mucosal: Epistaxis (nosebleed) or gingival bleeding
- Cutaneous: Petechiae, purpura, or ecchymoses
- Invasive sites that bleed longer than expected (injection sites, peripheral intravenous access sites)
- Occult or frank bleeding from any site, most notably the gastrointestinal tract or the genitourinary tract, respiratory tract, and/or the central nervous system
- Excessive menstrual bleeding

Practice Test Three

1.　You are supervising a nursing student who is caring for a patient who has just been diagnosed with myasthenia gravis. Which statement made by the nursing student to the patient will require correcting?

A. "Myasthenia gravis is an autoimmune disease."
B. "Myasthenia gravis often makes eating harder."
C. "Myasthenia gravis happens because the muscles are not able to receive impulses from the nerves like they should."
D. "Myasthenia gravis symptoms are the worst the during morning."

2.　You are caring for a patient who is recovering from a total knee arthroplasty three days ago who develops sudden shortness of breath, accompanied by chest pain and a blood-tinged cough. Which of the following conditions should be evaluated for first?

A. Pulmonary embolism
B. Cardiac tamponade
C. Myocardial infarction
D. Spontaneous pneumothorax

3.　What is the most common manifestation of coronary artery disease (CAD)?

A. Apnea
B. Weakness
C. Angina
D. Fluid retention

4.　An ACTH (adrenocorticotropic hormone) stimulation test is commonly used to diagnose:

A. Cystic fibrosis
B. Addison's disease
C. Grave's disease
D. Hashimoto's disease

5.   When caring for a female patient who will be undergoing a total proctocolectomy with ileostomy for her Crohn's disease, which of these comments made before surgery would indicate that she has concerns about her body image?

A. "I'm concerned that this may be only the first of many surgeries to come."
B. "I will have to discontinue my gym membership."
C. "I'm so afraid I may not survive the surgery."
D. "I need to go shopping for bigger, baggier clothing."

6.   A patient has a kidney stone that is composed of uric acid. Which of the following foods should the nurse instruct the patient to avoid?

A. Organ meats
B. Eggs
C. Fruits
D. Raw vegetables

7.   Which of the following transfusion reactions is most likely to occur with the administration of non-compatible blood?

A. Allergic reaction
B. Acute hemolytic
C. Transfusion-related acute lung injury (TRALI)
D. Febrile nonhemolytic

8.   You are providing teaching to a patient who has recently been diagnosed with multiple sclerosis. Which of the following statements best describes multiple sclerosis?

A. "Multiple sclerosis is known to be a progressive viral disease."
B. "Multiple sclerosis is a progressive disease that only affects motor neurons."
C. "Multiple sclerosis is a disease that causes degeneration of myelin sheaths."
D. "Multiple sclerosis may have remissions and exacerbations, but there is nothing that can be done to treat it."

9.   You are caring for a patient who is on 4 LPM of oxygen via nasal cannula. You understand that the percentage of the air that the patient breathes that is oxygen is approximately which of the following options?

      A. 53%
      B. 29%
      C. 37%
      D. 44%

10.   Important risk factors for heart failure include all of the following except:

      A. Hypertension
      B. Atherosclerotic disease
      C. History of heroin abuse
      D. Diabetes mellitus

11.   Traumatic pneumothorax occurs when trauma results in lung puncture, allowing air to pass into the pleural space. Which type of traumatic pneumothorax is due to blunt force, such as a car accident, fall, or fractured ribs?

      A. Open
      B. Iatrogenic
      C. Hemothorax
      D. Closed

12.   You are caring for a patient with type two diabetes mellitus. Which of the follow lab values would warrant further intervention?

      A. Anion Gap 8 mmol/L
      B. Hemoglobin A1C 8.9%
      C. Creatinine 0.5 mg/dL
      D. Glucose 112 mg/dL

13.   What is the primary symptom, and an early "red flag," of compartment syndrome following total joint arthroplasty (TJA)?

      A. Diminished pulses

B. Coolness of the affected extremity

C. Paresthesia

D. Increasing pain

14. You are caring for Mr. J, a patient receiving parenteral nutrition via a tunneled catheter (Broviac). Which of the following statements regarding this patient's care and treatment do you know to be true?

A. If this patient is willing to do so and his condition allows, he will be able to administer his nutrition at home

B. Dislodgement of the Broviac catheter is most likely to occur 3-4 weeks after placement

C. Broviac catheters may be inserted at the patient's bedside

D. Broviac catheters are most commonly placed in the basilic vein and advanced into the superior vena cava

15. Which of the following interventions is not indicated in a patient with paraplegia to help prevent pressure ulcers?

A. Encourage the patient to perform frequent active range of motion in all extremities

B. Avoid elevating the head of the bed beyond 30°

C. Use pillows to reduce pressure on bony prominences

D. Encourage adequate hydration and nutrition

16. Which of the following diagnostic studies is the most accurate measure of glomerular filtration rate (GFR)?

A. Urine sediment test

B. Urine creatinine clearance test

C. Urine osmolality test

D. Urinalysis

17.   You are caring for a 23-year-old male with complaints of passing out briefly multiple times in the last two months. He is lying in bed speaking to you when he suddenly stops responding to you. Which of the following actions should you take first?

A. Call a code blue
B. Check for a pulse
C. Perform a STAT EKG
D. Position the patient in the recovery position until he regains consciousness

18.   Corticosteroids are typically most beneficial for patients with respiratory disorders whose primary illness is:

A. Viral infections
B. Tuberculosis
C. Lung irritants such as tobacco smoke
D. Asthma

19.   Metabolic syndrome is identified by the presence of all of the following components except:

A. Fasting glucose greater than 100 mg/dL
B. Elevated blood pressure
C. Elevated waist circumference
D. Elevated HDL cholesterol

20.   Which of the following complications is of the greatest concern for someone who has experienced a compound fracture of the radius?

A. Contractures
B. Cellulitis
C. Osteomyelitis
D. Traumatic nerve damage

21. The most common complication of Peptic Ulcer Disease (PUD) is:

    A. Mid-epigastric pain
    B. Back pain
    C. Weight loss
    D. Gastrointestinal hemorrhage

22. Excessive collagen formation during healing is known as a:

    A. Bulla
    B. Keloid
    C. Telangiectasia
    D. Lichenification

23. Which of the following conditions most increases a patient's risk of chronic kidney disease?

    A. Lumbar spine fracture
    B. Gout
    C. Septic arthritis
    D. Osteoarthritis

24. The heart's electrical conduction network found within the ventricular myocardium is termed the:

    A. Atrioventricular (AV) node
    B. Purkinje fibers
    C. Sinoatrial (SA) node
    D. Bundle of His

25. The cardinal sign of respiratory disease is:

    A. Dyspnea
    B. Chest pain
    C. Cough
    D. Hemoptysis

26. Which of the following type 2 diabetes mellitus medications is to be taken with the very first bite of each meal?

   A. Sitagliptin (Januvia)
   B. Acarbose (Precose)
   C. Chlorpropamide (Diabinese)
   D. Dapagliflozin (Farxiga)

27. A patient with a fractured fibula is receiving skeletal traction and has external fixation in place. Which of the following do you instruct the nursing assistant to report immediately?

   A. The patient is complaining of pain and muscle spasm
   B. The patient wants to change position in bed
   C. The traction weights are resting on the floor
   D. There is a small amount of clear fluid on the skeletal pin sites

28. You are caring for Mr. H., who was admitted for an exacerbation of ulcerative colitis (UC). You gather the following data during your admission assessment:

   - Objective: Temperature: 101 degrees F, pulse 108, blood pressure: 101/55, respiratory rate: 20, O2 saturation: 98% room air
   - Subjective: frequent bloody stools, increased abdominal pain, decreased appetite with a 6-pound unexpected weight loss. noncompliance with pharmaceutical treatment plan due to financial restraints.

You anticipate that all of the following diagnostics and labs will be ordered on this patient except:

   A. Complete metabolic panel (CMP)
   B. Stool samples
   C. Serum amylase
   D. Complete blood count (CBC)

29. You are caring for a 35-year-old woman, in previous good health and on no medications, who was admitted to the hospital with petechiae mainly on her legs, hemorrhagic bullae of the oral mucosa, reddish to purple-colored spots and patches on the skin, epistaxis, and gingival bleeding. The only abnormal laboratory finding is a low platelet count of 30,000/mcL (normal is 150,000 to 400,000).

What is the most likely diagnosis?

A. Acute myelogenous leukemia (AML)
B. Idiopathic thrombocytopenia purpura (ITP)
C. Disseminated intravascular coagulation (DIC)
D. Multiple myeloma

30. This stone composition accounts for 75% of kidney stones:

A. Struvite
B. Cystine
C. Calcium
D. Uric acid

31. Which of the following is an example of an ACE inhibitor?

A. Metoprolol (Lopressor)
B. Amlodipine (Norvasc)
C. Amiodarone (Cordarone)
D. Captopril (Capoten)

32. All of the following are examples of antihistamines except:

A. Cetirizine (Zyrtec)
B. Fexofenadine (Allegra)
C. Guaifenesin (Mucinex)
D. Acrivastine (Semprex)

33. Which of the following symptoms is not a common genitourinary symptom of diabetes mellitus?

    A. Polycystic kidney disease
    B. Erectile dysfunction
    C. Bladder dysfunction
    D. Polyuria

34. Which of the following is not a risk factor for epilepsy?

    A. Alcohol use
    B. Cardiac arrhythmias
    C. Head trauma
    D. Genetics

35. Your patient has been prescribed an antacid for gastroesophageal reflux disease (GERD). You must instruct your patient to take this medication only as directed. If abused, what can occur?

    A. Diarrhea
    B. Systemic alkalosis
    C. Hypermagnesemia
    D. Constipation

36. Which of the following terms does not correctly describe psoriasis?

    A. Inflammatory
    B. Systemic
    C. Relapsing
    D. Chronic

37. Related to the genitourinary and reproductive systems of the geriatric patient, all of the following are typical physiologic changes except:

    A. Prostate gland enlargement, leading to urinary frequency
    B. Reduction in renal function and capacity
    C. Ovulation ceases and estrogen production decreases

D. Urinary incontinence

38. Which of the following is true about diastolic heart failure?

    A. A patient with diastolic heart failure will have a normal ejection fraction
    B. Diastolic heart failure will typically cause atrial fibrillation
    C. Unlike systolic heart failure, diastolic heart failure is not medically concerning
    D. Diastolic heart failure occurs when the ventricles are not able to fully empty as the heart pumps

39. The trachea branches into the right and left mainstream bronchi at the:

    A. Cricoid
    B. Carina
    C. Apex of the pleural cavity
    D. Apex of the diaphragm

40. In mild hypoglycemic reactions, when the patient has an intact swallowing response, which of the following should be given?

    A. 15 grams of protein
    B. 25 grams of protein
    C. 25 grams of fast-acting carbohydrates
    D. 15 grams of fast-acting carbohydrates

41. Which of the following statements is true related to range of motion (ROM)?

    A. ROM is the amount of motion available to a joint within the anatomic limits of its structure
    B. Passive ROM is typically assessed before active range of motion
    C. It is measured by grades
    D. If crepitus is encountered during ROM, passive manipulation of the joint must immediately cease

42. A patient with a recent ileostomy who is unable to toilet themselves tells you, "I think I just had a small bowel movement into my brief." What response is the most appropriate?

   A. "That was probably just gas. You may have more rectal gas after this surgery."
   B. "Let me check for you and see if you did."
   C. "Because you have an ileostomy, you will only have bowel movements into your bag for now."
   D. "Tell me more about how you feel about your body image now that you have had this surgery."

43. A patient presents with a skin infection caused by *Streptococcus pyogenes* (a group A beta-hemolytic bacterium). The patient's lower leg is infected from the deep dermis to the subcutaneous fat.

What skin disorder does this describe?

   A. Herpes zoster
   B. Varicella
   C. Psoriasis
   D. Cellulitis

44. The nurse knows that a female is at greater risk for developing cystitis than a male. What is the most common contributing factor to this increased risk?

   A. Hormonal secretions in females
   B. Shorter urethra in females
   C. Altered urinary pH in females
   D. Juxtaposition of the bladder in females

45. Which of the following patients is most at risk of developing endocarditis?

   A. A 17-year-old male with a history of asthma who underwent open thoracic surgery to repair a right lung bullet wound

B. A 65-year-old male with a dental abscess who has just undergone a hematopoietic stem cell transplantation

C. A 22-year-old female who has started heavily using marijuana concentrates over the last two months and was just involved in an MVC

D. A 91-year-old male who is unable to undergo a needed coronary artery bypass surgery due to severe heart failure

46. Your patient has been prescribed benzonatate (Tessalon). You conclude that the medication is having the intended effect if the patient experiences:

A. Decreased nausea and vomiting
B. Decreased frequency and intensity of cough
C. Decreased nasal congestion
D. Decreased pain

47. Which of the following organs is least likely to be affected by the pathology of diabetes mellitus?

A. Liver
B. Skin
C. Kidneys
D. Eyes

48. Which of the following is not a potential complication of brain attacks?

A. Tardive dyskinesia
B. Pressure ulcers
C. Spasticity
D. Increased intracranial pressure

49. Your patient has just returned to the medical-surgical floor from the post-anesthesia care unit following bowel resection surgery. To best prevent dehiscence, you should:

A. Make sure the patient is fully awake before offering fluids per mouth
B. Administer enoxaparin (Lovenox) as ordered

C. Remove the abdominal binder and encourage deep breathing every 2 hours

D. Keep the abdominal binder in place

50. Which of the following is considered the first-line treatment for idiopathic thrombocytopenia purpura (ITP)?

A. Platelet transfusion
B. Corticosteroids
C. Splenectomy
D. High-dose immunoglobulin therapy

51. Which of the following is not correct about acute pyelonephritis?

A. Acute pyelonephritis is typically accompanied by a fever
B. Acute pyelonephritis will cause irreversible renal damage in about 40% of cases
C. Acute pyelonephritis is usually caused by an infection
D. Pregnancy increases the risk of acute pyelonephritis

52. You are monitoring a patient with a junctional rhythm. You understand that with a junctional rhythm, which of the following is true?

A. The rhythm originates from the SA node
B. The rhythm can cause inverted T waves
C. The rhythm originates from the AV node
D. The rhythm can cause a QRS complex that is narrower than normal

53. The nurse is caring for a patient who has a chest tube connected to a wet system. The nurse is aware that:

A. The wall regulator controls the amount of suction in this system
B. Sterile water in the suction chamber typically turns blue
C. Continuous gentle bubbles should be seen in the water seal chamber
D. Continuous gentle bubbles should be seen in the suction chamber

54. Which of the following medications is not contraindicated in type 1 diabetes mellitus?

    A. Glimepiride (Amaryl)
    B. Metformin extended-release (Glucophage XR)
    C. Pramlintide (Symlin)
    D. Glipizide (Glucotrol)

55. Which of the following is the most appropriate nursing diagnosis for a patient with a strained ankle?

    A. Impaired physical mobility
    B. Risk for deficient fluid volume
    C. Disturbed body image
    D. Impaired skin integrity

56. Cardiopulmonary complications related to obesity include:

    A. Hypertension, elevated triglycerides, coronary artery disease
    B. Hypertension, hyperventilation syndrome, coronary artery disease
    C. Hyperventilation syndrome, elevated triglycerides, coronary artery disease
    D. Hypotension, hypoventilation syndrome, coronary artery disease

57. Which of the following is not part of the pathology of disseminated intravascular coagulation (DIC)?

    A. Increased blood pressure
    B. Increased blood clotting
    C. Increased bleeding
    D. Disruptions in blood circulation

58. The most common access to the circulatory system for chronic dialysis patients is:

    A. Arteriovenous (AV) fistula
    B. Central line catheter

C. Arteriovenous (AV) shunt

D. Peritoneal dialysis catheter

59. The conduction system is an electrical system that controls the heart rate, generates electrical impulses, and conducts them throughout the muscle of the heart, stimulating the heart to contract and pump blood. The sequence of travel by an action potential through the heart is:

A. Intra-atrial pathways, atrioventricular (AV) node, sinoatrial (SA) node, bundle of His, right and left branches, Purkinje fibers

B. Sinoatrial (SA) node, intra-atrial pathways, atrioventricular (AV) node, bundle of His, right and left branches, Purkinje fibers

C. Atrioventricular (AV) bundle, atrioventricular (AV) node, sinoatrial (SA) node, intra-atrial pathways, right and left branches, Purkinje fibers

D. Purkinje fibers, atrioventricular (AV) bundle, atrioventricular (AV) node, sinoatrial (SA) node, right and left branches, intra-atrial pathways

60. Of the following breath sounds, which may signify the need for emergency airway protection?

A. Stridor

B. Rhonchi

C. Crackles

D. Wheezes

61. This hormone inhibits the release of growth hormone (GH) and thyroid stimulating hormone (TSH) from the anterior pituitary gland:

A. Aldosterone

B. Corticotropin-releasing hormone

C. Gonadotropin-releasing hormone

D. Somatostatin

62. You are caring for a patient who has recently been diagnosed with rheumatoid arthritis who asks you what caused their condition. Which of the following responses is best?

    A. "Rheumatoid arthritis is caused by wearing down of the cartilage in your joints."
    B. "Rheumatoid arthritis occurs when your immune system attacks your joints."
    C. "Rheumatoid arthritis is caused by inflammation in the joints that sometimes occurs with the process of aging."
    D. "Rheumatoid arthritis occurs because of swelling in the joints that causes deformation, stiffness, and decreased circulation."

63. Which laxative promotes bowel movements by directly stimulating intestinal peristalsis?

    A. Psyllium (Metamucil)
    B. Docusate sodium (Colace)
    C. Bisacodyl (Dulcolax)
    D. Methylcellulose (Citrucel)

64. Which of the following four patients is at the greatest risk for developing pressure ulcers?

    A. A 67-year-old male with thrombocytopenia who has frequent diarrhea
    B. A 34-year-old male quadriplegic with new atrial fibrillation
    C. A 70-year-old female with gout who frequently asks for her PRN pain medications
    D. A 95-year-old female with pancreatitis who is able to perform her own ADLs

65. The nurse is teaching a male client to perform monthly testicular self-examinations. Which of the following points would be appropriate to make?

    A. Testicular cancer is a highly curable type of cancer
    B. Testicular cancer is very difficult to diagnose
    C. Testicular cancer is the number one cause of cancer death in males

D. Testicular cancer occurs most frequently in men over the age of 50

66. The nurse would expect to find which of the following test results in a patient just admitted with a diagnosis of heart failure?

A. Brain natriuretic peptide (BNP): elevated / Serum sodium: decreased
B. Brain natriuretic peptide (BNP): elevated / Serum sodium: elevated
C. Brain natriuretic peptide (BNP): decreased / Serum sodium: elevated
D. Brain natriuretic peptide (BNP): decreased / Serum sodium: decreased

67. A hospitalized patient with chronic obstructive pulmonary disease (COPD) is taking a bronchodilator and tells you that he is going to begin a smoking cessation program when he is discharged. You should tell the patient to notify the doctor if his smoking pattern changes because he:

A. May no longer need annual influenza immunizations
B. Will require an increase in antitussive medication
C. Will not derive as much benefit from inhaler use
D. May need his medication dosage adjusted

68. Which of the following eye disorders is not likely to be caused by the pathology of diabetes mellitus?

A. Glaucoma
B. Strabismus
C. Cataracts
D. Retinopathy

69. Which of the following terms is used to classify an immovable joint in which bones come into direct contact with each other?

A. Diarthrosis
B. Dysarthrosis
C. Amphiarthrosis
D. Synarthrosis

70. Acute gastrointestinal hemorrhage is characterized by which of the following clinical manifestations?

    A. Decreased platelet counts due to decreased coagulation process
    B. Body will attempt to expand plasma volume for 6-8 hours through the action of antidiuretic and aldosterone
    C. Decreased BUN as blood proteins are depleted
    D. Decreased creatinine level

71. Which of the following is not a type of burn?

    A. Convection burns
    B. Radiation burns
    C. Electrical burns
    D. Chemical burns

72. The nurse is assessing the urine of a patient with a urinary tract infection. Which of the following characteristic of the patient's urine should the nurse assess in each specimen?

    A. Specific gravity
    B. Viscosity
    C. Clarity
    D. Glucose

73. Assessing for distention of the neck veins can best be completed:

    A. With the patient sitting up at a 90-degree angle
    B. With the patient's head elevated 30-45 degrees
    C. With the patient in Trendelenburg position
    D. With the patient lying prone in bed

74. When performing an assessment on a patient with emphysema, you find that your patient has a barrel chest. The alteration in the patient's chest is due to:

    A. Hyperinflation of the lungs

B. Collapse of distal alveoli

C. Chronic hypoxia

D. Use of accessory muscles

75. Hashimoto's disease is:

A. A rare form of hypothyroidism

B. A form of hyperthyroidism

C. Chronic inflammation of the thyroid gland

D. Diagnosed most frequently in young adults

76. Which of the following statements is true related to osteoporosis?

A. Bisphosphonates are easily absorbed from the gastrointestinal tract

B. Calcium supplementation by itself is not a good treatment for osteoporosis

C. Calcitonin, available only in parenteral form, acts partly by blocking the effects of parathyroid hormone on bone resorption

D. Raloxifene (Evista) must be taken on an empty stomach

77. A patient is admitted to the hospital with severe pain, guarding, and rigidity of the abdomen. Labs indicate increased levels of amylase and leukocytosis. Cullen's sign is positive, and the patient is showing some signs of respiratory distress. The patient has a history of alcohol abuse. Which of the following conditions is most likely to be diagnosed?

A. Pneumonia

B. Alcoholic cirrhosis

C. Acute pancreatitis

D. Acute liver failure

78. The most common hematologic manifestation in Acquired Immune Deficiency Syndrome (AIDS) and a common complication of cancer and chemotherapy is:

A. Hemophilia

B. Polycythemia

C. Thrombocytopenia

D. Disseminated intravascular coagulation (DIC)

79. The diet which is most appropriate for the patient with glomerulonephritis includes all of the following except:

A. Low-potassium

B. Low-sodium

C. Low-calorie

D. Low-fluid

80. Cardiac effort that is effective in maintaining perfusion will be demonstrated by:

A. Systolic blood pressure greater than 80 mm/Hg

B. Skin that is cool and mottled

C. Mean arterial pressure less than 60 mm/Hg

D. A respiratory pattern that is eupneic

81. Which of the following is an untrue statement related to the upper airway?

A. The sinus cavities are not normally sterile

B. The sinuses assist in warming and humidifying inhaled air

C. The nose is composed of bones in the upper one-third

D. The oropharynx is the center for swallowing, serving as a pathway for air and food

82. A patient has recently undergone a total thyroidectomy. Which of the following findings warrants further investigation?

A. Creatinine 1.2 mg/dL

B. Potassium 3.5 mmol/L

C. Calcium 7.0 mg/dL

D. Sodium 135 mEq/L

83. Which of the following conditions does not increase the risk of an ischemic stroke?

    A. Atrial fibrillation
    B. Christmas disease
    C. Pregnancy
    D. Femur fracture

84. Which type of burn is characterized by damage resulting from heat made by a flowing current?

    A. Radiation burn
    B. Chemical burn
    C. Thermal burn
    D. Electrical burn

85. Which of the follow interventions will not help to prevent nephropathy caused by diabetes mellitus?

    A. Controlling hypertension
    B. Increasing dietary protein
    C. Controlling blood glucose levels
    D. Preventing urinary tract infections

86. Cardinal manifestations of heart failure include which of the following?

    A. Dyspnea, fatigue, pulmonary edema
    B. Rhonchi in lung fields, pulmonary edema, bradycardia
    C. Dyspnea, bradycardia, peripheral edema
    D. Ascites, bradycardia, dyspnea

87. You are caring for a patient who had surgical placement of a tracheostomy 48 hours ago due to his diagnosis of laryngeal cancer. What should your initial action be if the tube becomes dislodged?

    A. Ventilate the patient using a manual resuscitation bag while another nurse calls for help from the resuscitation team

B. Obtain the patient's vital signs

C. Re-insert the tube and notify the physician

D. Place a 4x4 sterile gauze over the stoma to prevent infection

88. Which of the following statements is true about type one diabetes mellitus?

   A. This type of diabetes is more likely to occur in people who are obese
   B. 80% of patients with this condition will require at least a below knee amputation (BKA) at some point in their lives
   C. Hyperosmolar hyperglycemic nonketotic syndrome (HHNS) is not a complication of this condition
   D. Insulin receptors become desensitized to insulin, creating elevated blood glucose levels

89. Which of the following is least likely to be a cause of rhabdomyolysis?

   A. Chest trauma
   B. Use of simvastatin (Zocor)
   C. Malignant hyperthermia
   D. Glomerulonephritis

90. You are caring for Mrs. M. who underwent an emergency gastric resection due to a perforated gastric ulcer. Postoperatively, she has a nasogastric tube (NG) in place to assist with stomach decompression and suction. All of the following are appropriate nursing interventions in caring for Mrs. M. except:

   A. Monitor for postoperative "dumping syndrome"
   B. Irrigate the NG tube every 8 hours
   C. Educate Mrs. M. to eliminate caffeine and spicy foods from her diet
   D. Monitor bowel sounds and flatus activity

91. You are caring for a patient who has a malignant melanoma. Which of the following is normally true about treatments for this condition?

   A. Treatment is primarily dependent on the diameter of the lesion
   B. Treatments are always palliative

C. Treatments are primarily often focused on slowing progression and relieving symptoms

D. Treatments for this will be primarily surgical and are often successful

92. Which of the following is not a complication of benign prostatic hypertrophy (BPH)?

A. Pyelonephritis
B. Bladder calculi
C. Urinary retention
D. Glomerulonephritis

93. Blood returning to the heart from the inferior vena cava would enter the:

A. Left ventricle
B. Right ventricle
C. Right atrium
D. Left atrium

94. You are caring for a patient who has emphysema. Which of the following statements by the patient indicates they understand your teaching on smoking cessation?

A. "I should cut the amount I smoke back by at least 75%."
B. "When I stop smoking, my emphysema will start to get better within a few months."
C. "Stopping smoking can help to slow or stop the progression of my emphysema."
D. "If I stop smoking, it will not help my breathing at all."

95. A patient with Cushing's disease is admitted to the medical-surgical unit. During the admission assessment, the nurse notes that the patient is agitated and irritable, has poor memory, reports loss of appetite, and appears disheveled. These findings are consistent with which problem?

A. Hypoglycemia
B. Neuropathy

C. Hyperthyroidism

D. Depression

96. The most common type of cartilage is:

   A. Fibrocartilage
   B. Elastic
   C. Cortical
   D. Hyaline

97. Which of the following is not an example of a proton pump inhibitor (PPI)?

   A. Omeprazole (Prilosec)
   B. Pantoprazole (Protonix)
   C. Rabeprazole (Aciphex)
   D. Famotidine (Pepcid)

98. The rule of nines must be modified for use in which of the following patients?

   A. A 70-year-old male with Parkinson's disease
   B. A 10-year-old female with muscular dystrophy
   C. An 18-year-old morbidly obese male
   D. A 38-year-old female with diabetes

99. The earliest presenting symptom of renal cell carcinoma is typically:

   A. Palpable flank mass
   B. Weight loss
   C. Hematuria
   D. Flank pain

100. Prior to auscultation of heart sounds, it is important to locate the auscultatory sites. Which of the following areas is located in the second right intercostal space?

    A. Mitral area or apex
    B. Pulmonic area
    C. Aortic area
    D. Tricuspid area

101. A patient is scheduled for a bronchoscopy. The nurse is aware that:

    A. This procedure allows for specimen collection via biopsy
    B. The patient should be informed of the warm, "flushed" feeling that may be experienced as dye is injected
    C. The patient will need to drink extra fluids following the procedure to help eliminate radioactive material
    D. The patient should have nothing by mouth for 24 hours prior to the procedure

102. Type 1 diabetes mellitus in both males and females typically presents during:

    A. Young adulthood
    B. Older adulthood
    C. Adolescence
    D. Childhood

103. All of the following statements are true related to osteoarthritis (OA) and the use of physical therapy except:

    A. Cardiovascular conditioning is important in patients with OA
    B. High-impact activities should be encouraged to improve joint strength
    C. Resistance exercises can contribute to decreased pain
    D. Weight-bearing exercises improve gait and overall function

104. You are assigned to care for Mrs. B., who was admitted to the medical-surgical unit with a 4-day history of nausea and vomiting. She has a medical history of chronic obstructive pulmonary disease, hypertension, and diabetes. She is weak and dehydrated. Many of her electrolytes are out of normal range. You complete a Malnutrition Screening Tool and calculate a score of 3.

Of the following, what is the best action to take next?

   A. Place a nutrition team screening consult in the patient's electronic chart
   B. Start an IV on the patient to replace fluids
   C. Inform the physician of your assessment findings
   D. Do a complete blood workup and place an abdominal CT order in the patient's electronic chart

105. Which of the following is not a risk factor for a sickle cell crisis?

   A. Iron deficiency
   B. Infection
   C. Dehydration
   D. Pregnancy

106. Which of the following conditions could be diagnosed using cystoscopy?

   A. Prostate cancer
   B. Pyelonephritis
   C. Kidney stones
   D. Bladder stones

107. The outer serous membrane of the wall of the heart is the:

   A. Myocardium
   B. Pericardium
   C. Epicardium
   D. Endocardium

108. Your patient is scheduled to have a pulmonary function test. You recognize further instruction is needed when the patient states:

    A. "This test will help identify the cause of my shortness of breath."
    B. "I should only breathe through my mouth."
    C. "I should use my albuterol right before the test."
    D. "I shouldn't smoke for 6 hours before the test."

109. Which of the following statements is true related to Graves' disease?

    A. It is the most common cause of adrenal insufficiency in adults
    B. It is the most common cause of hyperparathyroidism in adults
    C. It is the most common cause of hypothyroidism in adults
    D. It is the most common cause of hyperthyroidism in adults

110. Which of the following conditions is recognized as a central pain syndrome?

    A. Rheumatoid arthritis (RA)
    B. Fibromyalgia
    C. Systemic lupus erythematosus (SLE)
    D. Osteoarthritis (OA)

111. You are caring for a patient who was admitted to the medical-surgical unit with a diagnosis of cholecystitis caused by cholelithiasis. This condition typically manifests in individuals with consistently high:

    A. Blood glucose levels
    B. Liver enzymes
    C. Blood pressure
    D. Blood cholesterol levels

112. A patient who has sickle cell disease and does not yet have any children asks what the risk is that his children will have sickle cell disease. What response by the nurse is the best?

    A. "It will depend on who you have children with. You should avoid relationships with people who also have sickle cell disease."

B. "Your children will have sickle cell disease as well, and you should probably adopt instead of having children of your own."

C. "I can give you a referral to a genetic counselor who can discuss your children's risk with you."

D. "Sickle cell anemia is not a genetic disease, and your children will not be at increased risk because they are related to you."

113. The structure that contains the vas deferens and all arteries, veins, and lymph vessels that supply the testes is the:

A. Spermatic cord
B. Epididymis
C. Prostate gland
D. Seminal vesicle

114. Why are anticoagulants used for someone who has a deep vein thrombosis (DVT)?

A. To keep the DVT from growing
B. To promote the body's natural means of breaking down the thrombus
C. To reduce viscosity, promoting better circulation
D. To chemically degrade and break down the thrombus directly

115. The true vocal cords and the opening between them are called the:

A. Glottis
B. Vestibular folds
C. Cricoid cartilage
D. Thyroid cartilage

116. You are caring for a 45-year-old female with hyperthyroidism. Which of the following vital signs would you least expect to be elevated?

A. Oxygen saturation
B. Blood pressure
C. Respiratory rate
D. Temperature

117. Partial dislocation of a joint is known as:

    A. Ankylosis
    B. Contracture
    C. Kyphosis
    D. Subluxation

118. Which of the following statements is true related to Mallory-Weiss tears?

    A. They are treated with endoscopic therapy
    B. The risk of developing the condition is highly correlated with obesity
    C. They are often associated with diabetes
    D. They are treated preoperatively in an attempt to reduce the risk of cancer metastasis

119. You are reading the ER chart of a patient who is being admitted and note that the ER nurse wrote, "Telangiectasia noted on the right forearm." Which of the following should you expect related to this assessment when the patient arrives to your floor?

    A. The patient is likely on chemotherapy
    B. The patient has a liver problem that requires further assessment
    C. The patient may need steroids upon arrival
    D. The patient will not need any intervention for this finding

120. The glands that are responsible for influencing sodium levels, blood pressure, and water retention are:

    A. Parathyroid glands
    B. Bowman's glands
    C. Adrenal glands
    D. Prostate gland

121. The correct pathway that an erythrocyte would travel during systemic circulation is:

    A. Aorta > arteriole > capillary > venule > vein

B. Capillary > venule > vein > artery > aorta
C. Venule > vein > capillary > arteriole > aorta
D. Arteriole > aorta > vein > venule > capillary

122. Which of the following acid-base imbalances is probable in a patient who is hyperventilating?

A. Respiratory alkalosis
B. Metabolic acidosis
C. Metabolic alkalosis
D. Respiratory acidosis

123. A patient with central diabetes insipidus is ready for discharge on desmopressin (DDAVP). Which of the following instructions should the nurse provide?

A. "Your condition isn't chronic, so you won't need to wear a medical identification bracelet."
B. "You won't need to monitor your fluid intake and output after you start taking desmopressin."
C. "You may not be able to use desmopressin nasally if you have nasal discharge or blockage."
D. "Administer desmopressin while the suspension is cold."

124. Which of the following best describes meningitis?

A. An infection that causes headaches and confusion
B. A type of infectious bacteria
C. An inflammation of the tissues that line the brain and spinal cord
D. Any infection that affects the tissues of the brain

125. The most therapeutic diet for a patient being treated for hepatitis would include:

A. Increased calories with high protein, low carbohydrates, minimal fat
B. Increased calories with high protein, high carbohydrates, and minimal fat

C. Increased calories with low protein, high carbohydrates, minimal fat
D. Increased calories with high protein, high carbohydrates, high fat

126. Which symptom, if any, is expected in an otherwise healthy female patient with a hemoglobin of 10 g/dL?

A. Palpitations
B. Dyspnea
C. Pallor
D. None

127. Which of the following abnormal heart sounds is caused by incompetence of valves and/or abnormal blood flow patterns, and is most commonly described as a swishing or whooshing sound?

A. S3
B. Rub
C. Murmur
D. Gallop

128. The nurse assesses a male patient's respiratory status. Which of the following observations indicates that the patient is experiencing difficulty breathing?

A. Pursed-lip breathing
B. Diaphragmatic breathing
C. Use of accessory muscles
D. Controlled breathing

129. Symptoms of hypoglycemia related to the autonomic nervous system include all of the following except:

A. Tachycardia
B. Impaired thought processes
C. Tremors
D. Sweating

130.	You are caring for a patient who underwent a total left hip arthroplasty (THA) 8 hours ago. He is complaining of increasing, severe pain in the affected hip, despite receiving pain medication, and a tingling sensation in the left hip.

Which of the following complications do you suspect the patient is experiencing?

	A. Dislocation
	B. Infection
	C. Deep vein thrombosis (DVT)
	D. Compartment syndrome

131.	Mrs. S. has been admitted to the medical-surgical nursing unit with complaints of diffuse abdominal pain and distension that began one day ago. Your physical exam reveals that she has a temperature of 100.5 degrees F and her pulse is 133. She is diaphoretic and complains of chills. She is rating her pain as an "8" on a scale of 0-10. What is the most likely diagnosis?

	A. Cholecystitis
	B. Duodenal ulcer
	C. Peritonitis
	D. Inflammatory bowel disease (IBD)

132.	A patient is to receive epoetin (Epogen) injections. What laboratory value should the nurse assess before giving the injection?

	A. Prothrombin time (PT)
	B. Mean corpuscular hemoglobin concentration (MCHC)
	C. Activated partial thromboplastin time (APTT)
	D. Hematocrit (Hct)

133.	One of the responsibilities of a nurse in a fertility clinic is to provide health teaching to the patient in relation to the timing of intercourse. Patient instructions should include the information that the best time to achieve pregnancy is:

	A. Immediately after menses ends
	B. Midway between periods
	C. Fourteen days before the next period is expected

D. Fourteen days after the beginning of last period

134. You may see a slight increase in diastolic blood pressure early in some types of shock because:

A. Left ventricular contractions have strengthened
B. Concurrent brain injury is present
C. Stroke volume has increased
D. There is an increase in vascular tone

135. The most important factor for regulating respiratory rate is:

A. Oxygen levels in the cells
B. Bicarbonate level in the cells
C. Urea concentration in the blood
D. CO_2 level in the blood

136. Which of the following would be expected in a patient with primary hypothyroidism?

A. Increased TSH, increased T3/T4
B. Increased TSH, decreased T3/T4
C. Decreased TSH, increased T3/T4
D. Decreased TSH, decreased T3/T4

137. A patient was admitted to the medical-surgical unit complaining of difficulty holding objects. He states that his condition has progressively worsened. Based on the initial examination, the physician suspects Amyotrophic Lateral Sclerosis (ALS). The nurse is aware that characteristics of ALS include all of the following except:

A. Fasciculation of involved muscles
B. Memory loss
C. Dysphagia
D. Outbursts of uncontrolled crying

138. Which of the following diagnostic studies is the most reliable tool for gastrointestinal disorders?

    A. Ultrasonography
    B. Endoscopy
    C. Angiography
    D. Radiology

139. Which of the following cells produce antibodies?

    A. T cells
    B. Macrophages
    C. Leukocytes
    D. B cells

140. Conditions that stimulate the sympathetic nervous system (SNS) and lead to cardiac irritability include all of the following except:

    A. Anxiety
    B. Pain
    C. Hypoxia
    D. Vomiting

141. A postoperative patient who had a bronchoscopy two hours ago is NPO and states he is hungry. What should the nurse do?

    A. Order food for the patient
    B. Check for a gag reflex return
    C. Notify the physician
    D. Calmly tell the patient that he must remain NPO for at least 4 hours after the test

142. All of the following statements concerning exercise as it relates to diabetes mellitus are true except:

    A. Exercise enhances glucose transport into exercising muscle

B. The blood glucose-lowering effects of exercise occur during exercise and can persist for several hours following exercise

C. Exercise improves insulin sensitivity

D. Exercise can be effective in improving blood glucose control, especially in individuals with type 1 diabetes

143. Which of the following is not a potential complication of unilateral neglect following a brain attack?

A. Pressure ulcers

B. Hydrocephalus

C. Contractures

D. Deep vein thrombosis

144. All of the following consultations should be made for the patient except:

A. Gastroenterologist

B. Pain management

C. Nutritionist

D. Social Work

145. You are caring for a patient with neutropenia. Which of the follow is true about monitoring for potential infection?

A. Infections in neutropenic patients can be detected by sudden increases in white blood cell (WBC) counts

B. A low grade fever by itself is a cause for concern that there may be a severe infection

C. The only sign of infection in a patient with neutropenia may be pus production

D. Infection will not occur if reverse isolation precautions are followed

146. Which of the following is the location where fertilization occurs?

A. Ovaries

B. Fallopian tubes

C. Vagina

D. Uterus

147. When assessing your patient, you note a palpable precordial thrill. This finding may be caused by:

    A. Pulmonary edema
    B. Right ventricular hypertrophy
    C. Gallop rhythms
    D. Heart murmurs

148. You are discharging a patient who has been diagnosed with asthma. The patient asks you what potential triggers of asthma are. Which of the following would be incorrect?

    A. Inhaling perfume or cologne
    B. Humid air
    C. Emotional excitement or stress
    D. Exposure to cold

149. Neurological changes related to hyperthyroidism include all of the following except:

    A. Tremor
    B. Exophthalmos
    C. Heat intolerance
    D. Hyperreflexia

150. A patient is diagnosed with scoliosis with a spinal curve of 45 degrees. What is the recommended treatment?

    A. Surgery to correct spinal curvature
    B. Postural exercises
    C. Close monitoring every 6 months for disease progression
    D. Back bracing in the patient

Answer Key

Q.	1	2	3	4	5	6	7	8	9	10	11	12	13	14	15
A.	D	A	C	B	D	A	B	C	C	C	D	B	D	A	A

Q.	16	17	18	19	20	21	22	23	24	25	26	27	28	29	30
A.	B	B	D	D	C	D	B	B	B	A	B	C	C	B	C

Q.	31	32	33	34	35	36	37	38	39	40	41	42	43	44	45
A.	D	C	A	B	B	B	D	A	B	D	A	B	D	B	B

Q.	46	47	48	49	50	51	52	53	54	55	56	57	58	59	60
A.	B	A	A	D	B	B	C	D	C	A	A	A	A	B	A

Q.	61	62	63	64	65	66	67	68	69	70	71	72	73	74	75
A.	D	B	C	B	A	A	D	B	D	B	A	C	B	A	C

Q.	76	77	78	79	80	81	82	83	84	85	86	87	88	89	90
A.	B	C	C	C	D	A	C	B	D	B	A	A	C	D	B

Q.	91	92	93	94	95	96	97	98	99	100	101	102	103	104	105
A.	C	D	C	C	D	D	D	B	C	C	A	C	B	A	A

Q.	106	107	108	109	110	111	112	113	114	115	116	117	118	119	120
A.	D	C	C	D	B	D	C	A	B	A	A	D	A	D	C

Q.	121	122	123	124	125	126	127	128	129	130	131	132	133	134	135
A.	A	A	C	C	B	D	C	C	B	D	C	D	C	D	D

Q.	136	137	138	139	140	141	142	143	144	145	146	147	148	149	150
A.	B	B	B	D	D	B	D	B	B	B	B	D	B	B	A

Answers and Explanations

1.   D - Myasthenia gravis occurs because acetylcholine receptors are lost or blocked in neuromuscular junctions. Symptoms worsen with muscle use, making symptoms worse throughout the day. Symptoms will be least obtrusive in the morning and will worsen throughout the day.

2.   A - Prolonged immobility leads to an increased risk of thrombus development and is a risk factor for pulmonary embolism. The symptoms of pulmonary embolism include sudden shortness of breath, hemoptysis, and chest pain. Pulmonary embolism is a common complication post-surgery and is the third leading cause of death related to hospitalization.

3.   C - Coronary artery disease (CAD) develops when fat deposits (plaque) within the coronary arteries of the heart cause thickening and hardening of the artery walls and restrict blood flow. Angina, commonly referred to as "chest pain," occurs when oxygen delivery to the myocardium is decreased and is the *most* common manifestation of CAD.

4.   B - The ACTH stimulation test measures blood and urine cortisol before and after injection of ACTH. Patients with chronic adrenal insufficiency or Addison's disease generally do not respond with the expected increase in cortisol levels. An abnormal ACTH test may be followed by a CRH (corticotropin-releasing hormone) stimulation test to pinpoint the cause of adrenal insufficiency.

5.   D - Psychosocial support is necessary as a part of your nursing interventions regarding body image concerns. Body image refers to a person's perception of self and determines how the person interacts with others. The patient does not need to buy special clothing after ileostomy surgery, although some minor adjustments may be needed for comfort, such as stretch underwear or pantyhose for support.

6.   A - Uric acid stones accumulate due to the inefficient metabolism of purine proteins and are therefore controlled by a low-purine diet.

Foods that are high in purine are organ meats, meat extracts, shellfish, and red wines.

7. B - Acute hemolytic reactions occur because of the administration of non-compatible blood types.

8. C - Multiple sclerosis is a condition that causes degeneration of myelin sheaths that protect nerve axons. The exact cause of multiple sclerosis is unknown.

9. C - Oxygen makes up about 21% of the atmospheric gasses. When oxygen is applied via nasal cannula, each liter per minute equates to an increase of about 4% in the percentage of oxygen inspired. This means that a patient on 4 LPM of oxygen is breathing air that is approximately 37% oxygen (4 x 4% + 21% = 37%).

10. C - Heart failure (HF) is a complex clinical syndrome that results from any structural or functional impairment of ventricular filling or ejection of blood. History of heroin abuse is not a significant risk factor for HF.

11. D - Open pneumothorax is caused by impalement of an object into the chest cavity; iatrogenic results from an accidental puncture of the visceral pleura during the insertion of a central line, bronchoscopy, lung biopsy, or other medical procedure; and hemothorax (collection of blood in pleural space) often occurs with traumatic pneumothorax.

12. B - A normal A1C is 5.7-6.4%. A value of 8.9% would require intervention in the form or patient education or treatment modification.

13. D - Pain occurs as an early indicator of tissue compromise and should be recognized as a "red flag."

14. A - Tunneled catheters (Hickman, Broviac, and Groshong) are indicated when there is a need for central venous access for more than 4 weeks (longer-term) and are therefore a good choice for *home nutrition options*.

15. A - The patient's care plan should be tailored to his specific and unique situation. A patient who is paraplegic will be unable to perform active range of motion in his lower extremities, and this intervention will not work for this patient.

16. B - A urine creatinine clearance test measures a patient's urine over a 24-hour period, determining glomerular filtration rate as creatinine normally filters out in the glomerulus and is passed out of the system unchanged.

17. B - When a patient suddenly becomes unresponsive to verbal stimuli, checking for a pulse should be the first action you take.

18. D - Corticosteroids typically benefit individuals who have asthma as a respiratory issue.

19. D – The most widely used criteria for metabolic syndrome, characterized by a group of risk factors for cardiovascular disease and type 2 diabetes present in one person, are proposed by the U.S. Expert Panel on Detection, Evaluation, and Treatment of High Blood Cholesterol in Adults (Adult Treatment Panel III). This syndrome is identified by the presence of three or more of the following components:

    • Elevated waist circumference (men > 40 inches and women > 35 inches)
    • Elevated triglycerides (> 150 mg/dL)
    • Reduced (not elevated) HDL cholesterol (men < 40 mg/dL and women < 50 mg/dL)
    • Elevated blood pressure (> 130/85)
    • Fasting glucose > 100 mg/dL

20. C - Osteomyelitis is an infection of the bone and is commonly caused by compound fractures where the bone is potentially exposed to infectious organisms. Osteomyelitis requires immediate treatment and can lead to bone loss or amputation if it is not recognized and treated promptly.

21. D - Peptic Ulcer Disease (PUD) refers to an erosion of any portion of the GI tract and occurs when there is an imbalance between defensive resources and factors causing injury to the mucosal lining, such as gastric acid, hydrochloric acid, pepsin, or bile acids. GI hemorrhage is the most common complication of PUD; obstruction of the pyloric area due to edema and perforation are other less common complications of PUD.

22. B - Excessive collagen formation during healing is known as a keloid. This excessive tissue extends beyond the boundary of the wound and is irregular-shaped and elevated.

23. B - Gout causes increased levels of uric acid that must be filtered through the kidneys. This can lead to an increased risk of chronic kidney disease (CKD).

24. B - Normal excitation originates in the sinoatrial (SA) node (also known as the natural pacemaker), then propagates through both atria. The atrial depolarization spreads to the atrioventricular (AV) node, passes through the bundle of His, and then to the Purkinje fibers (found within the ventricular myocardium), which make up the left and right bundle branches; subsequently, all ventricular muscle becomes activated. Atrial and ventricular muscle masses are separate, and the conduction system is essential for coordination of their activity.

25. A - Dyspnea, or shortness of air (SOA), is the cardinal sign of respiratory disease. This is a subjective symptom; the description must be elicited from the patient.

26. B - Acarbose and Miglitol are alpha-glucosidase inhibitors. They improve glycemic control in adults with diabetes by slowing the breakdown of food absorption of sugar. They must be taken at the beginning of a meal to be effective.

27. C - When the traction weights are resting on the floor, they are not exerting pulling force to provide reduction and alignment, or to pre-

vent muscle spasm. The weights should always hang freely. Attending to the weights may reduce the patient's pain and spasm.

28. C - Serum amylase studies are not indicated for ulcerative colitis exacerbation, but rather in the diagnosis of pancreatitis.

29. B - ITP is considered a diagnosis of exclusion. All secondary causes of thrombocytopenia must be ruled out. In this case, routine workup shows normal findings.

30. C - Kidney stones are masses of crystals and proteins that obstruct urine flow. Calcium accounts for 75%-80% of kidney stones, including calcium phosphate and calcium oxalate stones.

31. D - Captopril, lisinopril, and enalapril are all examples of ACE inhibitors.

32. C - Guaifenesin is an expectorant and works by decreasing the viscosity of respiratory secretions to assist the bringing up of phlegm from the airways in acute respiratory tract infections.

33. A - Polycystic kidney disease is not a common genitourinary symptom of diabetes mellitus. Polyuria, erectile dysfunction, and bladder dysfunction are all common symptoms of diabetes mellitus.

34. B - Epilepsy is a seizure disorder in which the patient has had two or more unprovoked seizures. Cardiac arrhythmias are not a known risk factor for epilepsy.

35. B - Neutralizing agents, such as antacids, are commonly used in the treatment of GERD. Taking more than directed can lead to achlorhydria and systemic alkalosis.

36. B - Psoriasis is a skin condition in which skin cells grow too rapidly, causing plaques on the skin. Psoriasis may increase the risk of other conditions, such as arthritis, but it is not a systemic condition and only affects the skin. Psoriasis is a chronic condition. Relapses of psoriasis

can and do occur, interspersed with periods of remission. Psoriasis is an inflammatory condition.

37. D - Urinary incontinence is *not* a normal age-related change.

38. A - Diastolic heart failure occurs when the ventricles do not fill completely during diastole. Patients with diastolic heart failure will still have normal ventricular emptying, causing a normal ejection fraction.

39. B - It branches into right and left mainstream bronchi at the carina, which is approximately at the level of the sternal angle (angle of Louis).

40. D - In mild hypoglycemic reactions, when the patient has an intact swallowing response, the 15/15 rule is generally applied: eat 15 grams of fast-acting carbohydrates and wait 15 minutes.

41. A - ROM is measured in degrees, not by grades. In active ROM, the patient moves the joint, either independently or with minimal assistance (active assisted ROM); this is typically assessed first. In passive ROM, the examiner moves the joint while the patient's muscles are relaxed.

42. B - The nurse should not tell the patient they will only have bowel movements into their ostomy bag, as this may not be correct. The nurse should not dismiss the patient's statement, and increased rectal gas is not a consideration after having an ileostomy. While encouraging therapeutic expression is important, this does not address the patient's statement.

43. D - Cellulitis is a diffuse, acute bacterial infection of the skin and subcutaneous tissues usually caused by Group A beta-hemolytic streptococci or *Staphylococcus aureus*. It may also be caused by non-group A Streptococcus, *Haemophilus influenzae* type B, *Pseudomonas aeruginosa*, or *Campylobacter fetus*.

44. B - Cystitis is an inflammation of the bladder wall, often accompanied by urethritis. Because the female's urethra is much shorter than

the male's, bacteria may gain easier entry into the woman's bladder, causing infection.

45. B - Poor dentition and immunocompromised status are both risk factors for endocarditis. A patient who is undergoing hematopoietic stem cell transplantation has a highly compromised immune system at the time of the procedure.

46. B - Benzonatate (Tessalon) is a locally-acting (anesthetizes the stretch receptors) antitussive. Antitussives mostly suppress the cough center in the medulla of the brain. Its effectiveness is measured by the degree to which it decreases the intensity and frequency of coughing without eliminating the cough reflex.

47. A - Diabetes mellitus can lead to kidney damage, retinopathy, and neuropathy that leads to impaired skin integrity. The liver is typically the least affected of the four organs mentioned.

48. A - Tardive dyskinesia causes repetitive and involuntary movement and is often the result of the long-term use of psychiatric medications. Tardive dyskinesia is not caused by brain attacks and is not a potential complication.

49. D - Dehiscence (wound ruptures along a surgical incision) is a serious surgical complication, especially with abdominal incisions, which may occur when sutures start to give way and may be caused by infection, marked abdominal distention, strenuous coughing, increasing age, and poor nutritional status. It is best prevented by using and keeping an abdominal binder in place.

50. B - In ITP, if the patient is asymptomatic, intervention may not be warranted until platelet count falls below 30,000. Once warranted, prednisone is the first-line treatment to decrease antibody formation, suppress platelet destruction by macrophages in the spleen, decrease fragility and bleeding time, and increase the lifespan of platelets; 80% of patients treated will see platelet counts return to normal within 1-3 weeks.

51. B - While chronic pyelonephritis may cause long-term, irreversible renal damage, acute pyelonephritis rarely does.

52. C - Junctional rhythms originate from the AV node, not the SA node. Junctional rhythms do not cause changes to the QRS complex. Junctional rhythms can cause inverted P waves, not inverted T waves.

53. D - Continuous gentle bubbles *should not* be seen in the water seal chamber (this could indicate an air leak). Sterile water is used to fill the water seal chamber (not the suction chamber), which typically turns blue in most systems. It is the amount of water in the suction chamber that controls the amount of suction, not the wall regulator.

54. C - Pramlintide is an amylin analog. It is used to control blood sugar in people with type 1 and type 2 diabetes mellitus (DM). This medicine is always used with insulin.

55. A - Ankle strains result in pain and damage to the muscle body and tendon (from overstretching, misuse, or overexertion), as well as altered physical mobility.

56. A - Complications related to obesity are multisystemic. By system, these complications include:

    • Cardiopulmonary: hypertension, elevated triglycerides, coronary artery disease, hypoventilation syndrome
    • Musculoskeletal: arthritic conditions, gout
    • Gastrointestinal: GERD, fatty liver (can result in liver failure), gallstones
    • Endocrine: diabetes mellitus due to hyperinsulinemia and insulin resistance
    • Other complications associated with obesity include an increased risk for cancer and psychosocial complications including social stigma/discrimination and depression.

57. A - Increased blood pressure is not part of the pathology of DIC.

58.   A - The AV fistula is the most common access route for chronic dialysis patients; it is a surgically created internal passageway between an artery and a vein and is considered the gold standard for long-term hemodialysis access.

59.   B - Electrical signals arising in the SA node (located in the right atrium) stimulate the atria to contract and travel to the AV node (through the intra-atrial pathways). After a delay, the stimulus diverges and is conducted through the left and right bundle of His to the respective Purkinje fibers for each side of the heart, as well as to the endocardium at the apex of the heart, then finally to the ventricular epicardium.

60.   A - Stridor is a high-pitched inspiratory sound associated with upper airway obstruction. It is usually heard when taking in a breath and may signify the need for emergency airway protection. One common cause of stridor is croup (a viral respiratory infection), most commonly seen in children.

61.   D - Somatostatin, also called the growth hormone-inhibiting hormone (GHIH), acts as an important regulator of endocrine and nervous system function by inhibiting the anterior pituitary gland's secretion and release of GH and TSH.

62.   B - Rheumatoid arthritis is an autoimmune condition in which the body's immune system attacks tissues in the joint, leading to pain, deformity, and limited range of motion.

63.   C - Stimulants, such as bisacodyl (Dulcolax), promote bowel movements by directly stimulating intestinal peristalsis.

64.   B - A patient with quadriplegia will have limited mobility and incontinence, two significant risk factors for pressure ulcers. Additionally, he will be unable to reposition himself, further increasing his risk.

65.   A - Testicular cancer is highly curable, particularly when it is treated in its early stage; it is most often unilateral and has a 95% cure rate.

66. A - Brain natriuretic peptide (BNP) is an endogenous chemical released in response to elevated pulmonary capillary pressure. Increased BNP levels in the serum are used as markers of severity in heart failure. Dilutional hyponatremia (decreased sodium levels) is also seen, as heart failure impairs the ability to excrete ingested water by increasing antidiuretic hormone (ADH) levels.

67. D - Changes in smoking patterns should be discussed with the physician because they have an impact on the amount of medication needed.

68. B - Strabismus is when the eyes do not align with each other when looking at an object and is not related to diabetes.

69. D - An immovable joint in which bones come into direct contact with each other is known as synarthrosis. The bones are separated only by a thin layer of fibrous connective tissue; cranial suture joints are an example.

70. B - Gastrointestinal hemorrhage is defined as acute loss of blood from the upper GI tract. "Acute" or "massive" bleeding is defined as loss of 25% of circulating volume (approximately 1,500 mL in adults). Clinically, the patient's body will attempt to expand plasma volume due to the action of antidiuretic and aldosterone

71. A - While convection may transfer heat, the method by which the heat is transferred is not a type of burn, and these burns would be considered thermal burns. Convection burns are not recognized as a type of burn.

72. C - Urine that is cloudy indicates purulent drainage that is associated with an infection.

73. B - During inspection, observing for neck vein distention (a sign of peripheral vascular disease) can best be visualized *with the patient's head elevated at 30–45 degrees.*

74. A - Patients with emphysema develop a barrel chest due to obstruc-

tions in the passages that deliver air to the lung tissue. Air gets trapped within the lung and causes alveoli to become enlarged and lungs to become overinflated.

75. C - Hashimoto's disease is the most common cause of hypothyroidism. It is an autoimmune disease that produces chronic inflammation of the thyroid gland (thyroiditis).

76. B - Adequate calcium is important to bone health but is not a treatment for osteoporosis. Supplementation with vitamin D may be necessary to maximize absorption for patients who do not get enough sun exposure.

77. C - Patients with acute pancreatitis clinically present as acutely ill, with severe pain, guarding, and rigidity of the abdomen. Labs indicate increased amylase and leukocytosis (increased white blood cells). The incidence of acute pancreatitis is 1/10,000 in the general population; 1/100 among alcoholics.

78. C - Thrombocytopenia is defined as a decrease in the number of circulating platelets to less than 100,000 to 150,000 per microliter of blood; this is the most common hematologic manifestation in AIDS, and there is a decreased production of precursor platelets by bone marrow in hematologic cancers and chemotherapy.

79. C - Education for the patient with glomerulonephritis about the importance of a high-calorie, low-protein, low-sodium, low-potassium, low-fluid diet is imperative to ensure adequate caloric intake, without promoting further fluid retention or hyperkalemia.

80. D - Eupnea (normal, unlabored respirations at a rate of 10-20 breaths/minute) is a sign of adequate cardiac effectiveness.

81. A - The sinuses (frontal, maxillary, ethmoid, sphenoid) surround the nasal cavity and assist in warming and humidifying inhaled air; they normally *are sterile*.

82.   C - A low calcium level (normal 8.6-10.3 mg/dL) can indicate that the parathyroid glands were affected during the patient's surgery and would warrant further investigation. The other three values are normal and do not require any further intervention.

83.   B - Christmas disease, also called hemophilia B, is a disorder where a clotting factor IX deficiency increases the risk of bleeding. This condition does not increase the risk of an ischemic stroke.

84.   D - The causes of burns include thermal, chemical, electrical, and radiation. *Electrical burns* are damage resulting from heat made by flowing current. The nerves and blood vessels are very good conductors in this type of burn, and electrical current travels through most conductive tissue.

85.   B - Decreasing, not increasing, dietary protein will help to prevent nephropathy caused by diabetes mellitus.

86.   A - Cardinal manifestations of heart failure are dyspnea and fatigue, which may limit exercise tolerance, and cause fluid retention leading to pulmonary edema and/or peripheral edema.

87.   A - Tube dislodgement that occurs within 72 hours after surgery is an emergency. As such, ventilating the patient *first* is a priority, followed by the other options. Always remember your ABCs. (Airway, breathing, circulation)

88.   C - While diabetic ketoacidosis (DKA) is a complication of type one diabetes, HHNS is specific to only type two diabetes.

89.   D - Rhabdomyolysis is the breakdown of muscle tissue and can lead to kidney failure if not treated. While rhabdomyolysis can cause kidney damage, glomerulonephritis is not a cause of rhabdomyolysis.

90.   B - Irrigate the NG tube *only with a physician order, due to the risk of injuring the anastomotic site.* NG tubes that are used for suction are not

routinely irrigated and will not normally be irrigated unless they are obstructed and there are no contraindications to irrigating.

91. C - Malignant melanoma often has a poor prognosis and there are no dependable, curative, systemic treatments for malignant melanoma. Treatments are often primarily focused on slowing progression and relieving symptoms, not curing the disease. Treatments are multifaceted and not always palliative.

92. D - Glomerulonephritis is inflammation of the glomeruli and is not caused by infections or changes in the urinary tract.

93. C - Blood flow through the heart: vena cava (superior or inferior) > right atrium > right ventricle through tricuspid valve > pulmonary artery through pulmonic valve > lungs > pulmonary vein > left atrium > left ventricle through mitral valve > aorta through aortic valve

94. C - Smoking cessation will not help to reverse emphysema, but can help to stop or slow its progression.

95. D - Agitation, irritability, poor memory, loss of appetite, and neglect of one's appearance may signal depression, which is common in patients with Cushing's disease.

96. D - Hyaline (transparent) cartilage is the most common type of cartilage; it covers joint surfaces to reduce friction as adjacent bones slide over each other during movement; it is also found in the trachea, larynx, and nose. It has a considerable amount of collagen and contains no nerves or blood vessels.

97. D - Famotidine (Pepcid) is a histamine blocker (H_2 receptor antagonist), not a proton pump inhibitor (PPI). It works by blocking the action of histamine at the H_2 receptors of the parietal cells in the stomach and decreasing hydrogen ion production, which in turn increases stomach pH, providing symptom relief.

98. B - The rule of nines gives a quick estimation of burn size in a patient.

It must be modified for use in *children less than 15 years of age* because it does not accurately reflect body surface area.

99. C - Renal cell carcinoma is a malignant renal neoplasm. Only 10% of cases present with symptoms that represent advanced stage. Hematuria (presence of red blood cells in the urine) is the most common and earliest presenting symptom of renal cell carcinoma.

100. C - The *aortic area* of the heart is generally auscultated in the second right intercostal space (ICS), near the sternum.

101. A - A bronchoscopy permits direct visualization of the larynx, trachea, and bronchi, and allows for specimen collection via biopsy, brushes, or washes.

102. C - Peak incidence of type 1 diabetes mellitus (DM) in both men and women is in adolescence and may require counseling on weight issues and insulin dosing.

103. B - Physical therapy for the patient with osteoarthritis focuses on cardiovascular conditioning, improved strength and flexibility, and increased joint mobility.

104. A - Being a proactive nurse, you should *first* place a nutrition team screening consult/referral in the electronic medical record because you know a score of 2 or greater suggests malnutrition. Next, you should inform the physician of your assessment findings and follow-up referral that you placed.

105. A - Sickle cell crisis occurs when hemoglobin interacts with other hemoglobin in the red blood cells, forming long, rigid chains that cause the red blood cells to change into a crescent or sickle shape.

106. D - A cystoscopy involves using an endoscope to visualize the bladder and urethra. Bladder stones can be visualized and diagnosed using cystoscopy.

107. C - The wall of the heart consists of three layers: Endocardium: inner lining, myocardium: middle layer, and epicardium: outer serous layer.

108. C - Patients are to avoid smoking or use of bronchodilators for 6 hours before testing; albuterol is a bronchodilator that must be withheld 6 hours before the procedure as not to skew the results.

109. D - Graves' disease is an autoimmune disorder characterized by an enlarged thyroid gland and overproduction of thyroid hormones. It produces symptoms of hyperthyroidism such as tachycardia, palpitations, arrhythmias, heat intolerance, agitation or irritability, weight loss, and trouble sleeping.

110. B - Fibromyalgia is a connective tissue disorder now recognized as one of the central pain syndromes; it may coexist with other inflammatory diseases, such as rheumatoid arthritis or systemic lupus erythematosus.

111. D - Cholecystitis is inflammation of the gallbladder, usually caused by the presence of gallstones (cholelithiasis). Stone development usually occurs in people with consistently high blood cholesterol levels.

112. C - Referring the patient to a genetic counselor who can discuss the issue more in depth is the appropriate action. The patient's risk of having children who have sickle cell disease is dependent on if he has children with someone who has sickle cell disease or is a carrier for sickle cell disease.

113. A - The spermatic cord contains the vas deferens and all arteries, veins, and lymph vessels that supply the testes.

114. B - Unlike thrombolytic medications, anticoagulants do not break down thrombi directly. While anticoagulants will help DVTs from growing, that is not the main reason for their use in patients who already have a DVT. Anticoagulants do not meaningfully contribute to blood viscosity and are not used for this purpose.

115. A - The glottis, located between the vocal cords, opens into the trachea and is important for effective coughing.

116. A - Hyperthyroidism leads to increased metabolism and speeds up most body systems. This leads to an elevated temperature, respiratory rate, and blood pressure. The patient's oxygen saturation will be unaffected.

117. D - Dislocation occurs when one or more bones of the joint are out of position; the articulating surfaces of the joint lose contact. When the surfaces partially lose contact, it is known as subluxation.

118. A - Mallory-Weiss tears are esophageal tears in the gastric mucosa at the esophagogastric junction probably due to mechanical irritation such as forceful vomiting; there is a strong correlation with alcohol and aspirin abuse. They are treated with endoscopic therapies including ligation, cauterization, embolization, and intra-arterial infusion of vasopressin.

119. D - Telangiectasia is a skin lesion that is characterized by fine, irregular lines. This skin condition is benign and is not typically an indicator of any concerning disease process.

120. C - The adrenal glands are located at the top of each kidney and influence sodium and water retention, as well as regulation of blood pressure.

121. A - The peripheral vascular system functions by maintaining blood flow to supply tissues throughout the body with adequate oxygen and nutrients; it carries oxygenated blood away from the heart to the body, and returns deoxygenated blood back to the heart. Blood flow through systemic circulation is as follows: heart > arteries > arterioles > capillaries > venules > veins > heart.

122. A - Respiratory alkalosis occurs when the blood becomes more basic (less acidic) due to the influence of the respiratory system. It typically results from expiring too much carbon dioxide, reducing the acidity of the blood, and raising the pH.

123. C - Desmopressin may not be absorbed if the intranasal route is compromised; it can also be taken orally or injected subcutaneously or intravenously.

124. C - Meningitis is an inflammation of the meninges, the tissues that line the brain and spinal cord.

125. B - Instruct the patient that fat in the diet needs to be as minimal as tolerated to allow the liver to rest. The patient needs adequate intake of both protein and carbohydrates and these should not be restricted. Vitamin B and vitamin K supplements should be added. The patient should also be instructed to abstain from alcohol and drugs.

126. D - Normal hemoglobin values for females range from 12 to 16 g/dl. A hemoglobin of 10 g/dl would be mild anemia, which usually has no clinical signs or symptoms.

127. C - A murmur is heard with a stethoscope upon auscultation. Although most murmurs are innocent and don't require treatment, the clinical nurse is not expected to interpret abnormal heart sounds, but rather identify them correctly and inform the physician of their presence.

128. C - The use of accessory muscles for respiration indicates the patient is having difficulty breathing.

129. B - Symptoms of hypoglycemia related to the *autonomic* nervous system include: tachycardia, tremors, palpitations, nausea, sweating, and hunger.

130. D - Compartment syndrome is a medical emergency marked by the development of high pressure in a muscle compartment in closed fascial space; it is related to swelling, and can occur within 6-8 hours after surgery or may take up to 2 days to manifest, with decreased circulation as a result.

131. C - Peritonitis is defined as inflammation within the peritoneum and occurs when intestinal contents or bacteria enter the sterile peritone-

um, initiating an inflammatory response and resulting in chemical or bacterial infection with subsequent peritoneal fluid shift and ultimately shock if not corrected.

132. D - Epoetin (Epogen) is a biosynthetic form of the endogenous erythropoietin, which stimulates red blood cell (RBC) production in the bone marrow and therefore causes the hematocrit to rise. The elevation in hematocrit causes an elevation in blood pressure.

133. C - Ovulation generally occurs 14 days before the onset of menses.

134. D - An increase in vascular tone (constricting the vessels) results in an increase in diastolic blood pressure. This is seen in compensated shock and results in a narrowing of the pulse pressure.

135. D - Small changes in the $PaCO_2$ in the systemic arterial blood flowing to the medulla produce pronounced changes in ventilation; thus, CO_2 is the single most important factor for regulation of respiratory rate.

136. B - Levels of the thyroid hormones T3 and T4 will be decreased with primary hypothyroidism, while the thyroid stimulating hormone (TSH) will be elevated as the body attempts to stimulate the production of more thyroid hormones.

137. B - ALS is a progressive, degenerative disease involving the destruction of the motor neurons of the anterior horn cells (in the spinal cord), brainstem (especially cranial motor nerves), and cerebral cortex. Cognitive problems such as memory loss are not present in ALS.

138. B - Endoscopy is one of the most reliable diagnostic tools for gastrointestinal disorders because it can pinpoint the area of concern. A flexible, lighted tube called an endoscope is inserted orally or rectally for *direct* visualization of the concerning area of the GI tract.

139. D - Leukocytes are simply white blood cells (WBCs); B cells are a type of WBC, known as B lymphocytes, that produce antibodies.

While B cells are technically a type of leukocyte, not all leukocytes produce antibodies.

140. D - Anxiety and stress, pain, hypoxia, and fear all stimulate the SNS, which leads to cardiac irritability. Vomiting, the Valsalva maneuver, and carotid receptor stimulation all activate the *parasympathetic nervous system* (PNS), leading to cardiac depression.

141. B - The anesthesia from bronchoscopy inhibits swallowing. Therefore, it is important for the nurse to check for the gag reflex as an aspiration precaution before allowing the patient to eat.

142. D - Regardless of whether the person has diabetes type 1 or type 2, the benefits of exercise are extremely important. The blood glucose-lowering effects of exercise occur during exercise and can persist for several hours following exercise. Exercise improves insulin sensitivity and enhances glucose transport into the exercising muscle(s).

143. B - Hydrocephalus is swelling in the ventricles of the brain. While hydrocephalus is a potential complication of a brain attack, is not a complication that is associated with unilateral neglect.

144. B - Pain management is not generally necessary as symptoms can be well managed with drug therapies consisting of aminosalicylates, antimicrobials, corticosteroids, immunosuppressants, and biologic therapy.

145. B - A patient with neutropenia will have a blunted immune response, and a low grade fever may be the only indicator that a severe infection is developing.

146. B - The fallopian tubes are bilateral ducts that enter the uterus on either side; they conduct ova via peristalsis from the space around the ovary to the uterus, and fertilization usually occurs here, in the distal two-thirds of the tube (ampulla).

147. D - The precordium is located between the apex and sternum. Normally, no pulsations are seen or felt here. However, if abnormal pal-

pable vibrations or pulsations are present, (called thrills), they may be indicative of heart murmurs, which are caused by incompetence of valves and/or abnormal blood flow patterns.

148. B - Humid air may be an indirect trigger of asthma in that it may create an environment where triggers such as mold exist. Humid air may also be more prone to retaining pollutants that may trigger asthma. Humid air itself, however, is not an asthma trigger.

149. B - Hyperthyroidism is a disorder of the thyroid gland in which there is a hypersecretion of thyroid hormones. Neurological changes related to hyperthyroidism include: tremor, excessive sweating, hyperreflexia, and heat intolerance

150. A - Surgery is generally recommended for curves greater than 40 degrees. Surgical options include anterior or posterior spinal fusion, or combined anterior and posterior surgery as a staged procedure.

Practice Test Four

1. The physician has ordered an oral cholecystogram for your patient. All of the following nursing actions are appropriate in preparing the patient for this procedure except:

   A. Administer radiopaque dye orally
   B. Administer a fat-free meal the evening before the test
   C. Allow the patient to drink water after administration of radiopaque dye
   D. Determine sensitivity to iodine

2. You are caring for a patient who was admitted to the hospital to rule out pernicious anemia, a deficiency of vitamin B12. You recognize that the primary problem associated with this condition occurs due to a lack of intrinsic factor (IF) secreted from the stomach, which is required to:

   A. Produce vitamin B12
   B. Digest vitamin B12
   C. Store vitamin B12
   D. Absorb vitamin B12

3. This structure transports sperm to the urethra:

   A. Mons pubis
   B. Prostate
   C. Vas deferens
   D. Cowper's glands

4. You are caring for a patient who is in acute renal failure (ARF) who asks about his continuing treatment and prognosis. Which of the following statements to the patient is correct?

   A. "Everyone who has acute renal failure needs to be on dialysis until it resolves."
   B. "You will need a intravenous pyelogram to evaluate the blood flow in your kidneys."

C. "You will need a medication called Lasix during the oliguric phase of acute renal failure."

D. "Acute renal failure is often reversible."

5. Which of the following might lead you to consider obstructive shock over hypovolemic shock?

A. Widening pulse pressure
B. Suspicion of significant closed head injury
C. Distended neck veins
D. Indications of abdominal injury

6. The parietal pleural membrane lines the inside of the:

A. Pulmonary artery
B. Thoracic cavity
C. Abdominal cavity
D. Lungs

7. All of the following are examples of rapid-acting insulins except:

A. Levemir (Detemir)
B. Novolog (Aspart)
C. Apidra (Glulisine)
D. Humalog (Lispro)

8. While assessing a patient recently diagnosed with rheumatoid arthritis (RA), the nurse should expect to find:

A. Fibrosis of joints
B. Mild heart murmur
C. Deformed joints of the hand
D. Early morning stiffness

9. A patient with severe variceal bleeding is to undergo a transjugular intra-hepatic portosystemic shunt. The nurse is explaining the procedure to the patient's family. She tells the family:

   A. The advantage of this procedure is that it can be performed in the interventional radiology department
   B. Another name for this procedure is the Billroth II
   C. This procedure is sometimes called a portacaval shunt
   D. A common side effect of this procedure is dumping syndrome

10. A patient who was tested for human immunodeficiency virus (HIV) after a recent exposure had a negative result. During the post-test counseling session, you should tell the patient which of the following?

    A. This negative result ensures that the patient is not infected with HIV
    B. The test should be repeated in 3 months
    C. The patient likely has immunity to the acquired immunodeficiency virus
    D. The patient no longer needs to use protection during sexual encounters

11. The normal range for cardiac output is:

    A. 12-16 L/min
    B. 16-20 L/min
    C. 8-12 L/min
    D. 4-8 L/min

12. All of the following statements related to sputum specimens are correct except:

    A. Only a single specimen is required for culturing to identify pulmonary infections
    B. Broad spectrum antibiotics should started initially until a specimen can be collected
    C. Sputum specimens can be used to identify cancer cells
    D. The specimen must come from the lung, not from the oropharynx

13. You are caring for a patient with type 1 diabetes mellitus who exhibits confusion, light-headedness, and impaired thought processes and has a bedside blood glucose level of 52. The patient is still conscious. You should first administer:

   A. 15 grams of a fast-acting carbohydrate such as orange juice
   B. IM or SQ glucagon
   C. 10 units of fast-acting insulin
   D. IV bolus of dextrose 50%

14. You are caring for a patient who has just been diagnosed with Parkinson's disease. Which of the following statements made to the patient would be correct?

   A. "This disease occurs because you produce too much dopamine."
   B. "Parkinson's disease may cause you to develop joint or muscular pain."
   C. "You will start to slowly lose your ability to move until you are completely paralyzed."
   D. "Parkinson's disease may cause a deteriorating quality of life, but it is not deadly."

15. You are providing discharge teaching to a patient who was admitted for peptic ulcer disease (PUD). Which of the following statements by the patient indicates the need for further teaching?

   A. "I should try to take Tylenol instead of Aleve for my joint pain."
   B. "If I stop smoking, it will reduce my risk of peptic ulcer disease in the future."
   C. "Stress reduction will help me to avoid having worsening of my peptic ulcer disease."
   D. "Peptic ulcer disease is never caused by infections."

16. Which of the following statements related to basal cell carcinoma is true?

   A. Growth rate of a basal cell tumor is rapid
   B. It has a high rate of metastasis
   C. It is the primary cause of death of all skin diseases
   D. It has a low rate of metastasis

17.   Accuracy of a pregnancy test in detecting human chorionic gonadotropin (HCG) in urine is greatest:

A. 6 weeks after last menstrual period
B. 4 weeks after last menstrual period
C. 8 weeks after last menstrual period
D. 10 weeks after last menstrual period

18.   Which of the following routes is not used to administer nitroglycerin in treating cardiac ischemia?

A. Topically
B. Subcutaneously
C. Sublingual
D. Intravenously

19.   The lower airway consists of the:

A. Trachea, lungs, and alveoli
B. Trachea and lungs
C. Bronchial airway and lungs
D. Pulmonary artery and lungs

20.   Addison's disease involves destruction of the:

A. Parathyroid gland
B. Adrenal medulla
C. Hypothalamus gland
D. Adrenal cortex

21.   Which of the following terms is used to classify an immovable joint in which bones come into direct contact with each other?

A. Diarthrosis
B. Dysarthrosis
C. Amphiarthrosis
D. Synarthrosis

22. Complications of gastroesophageal reflux disease (GERD) include all of the following except:

   A. Barrett's esophagus
   B. Asthma and cough
   C. Esophageal varices
   D. Esophagitis

23. Which immune cell is responsible for the quickest release of histamine that causes the red, itchy welts associated with allergies?

   A. Basophil
   B. Lymphocyte
   C. Eosinophil
   D. Mast cell

24. Most cases of acute pyelonephritis are caused by:

   A. *Klebsiella* invasion
   B. Fungal or viral infections
   C. *Proteus* invasion
   D. *Escherichia coli* invasion

25. Which of the following statements is true related to cardiac valvular disorders?

   A. Rheumatic fever is the most common cause of valvular disorders worldwide
   B. Valve stenosis refers to the inability of the valve to completely close
   C. Mitral insufficiency is more common in women than in men
   D. Left ventricular hypertrophy is associated with mitral stenosis

26. You are caring for a patient with chronic obstructive pulmonary disease (COPD). You notice that the patient demonstrates more dyspnea in certain positions. Which position is most likely to alleviate the patient's dyspnea?

    A. Lying with head slightly lowered
    B. Standing or sitting upright
    C. Side-lying with the head of the bed elevated
    D. Lying supine with a single pillow

27. Which of the following complications can occur from electrolyte shifts caused by IV insulin therapy for a patient in diabetic ketoacidosis?

    A. Decreased glomerular circulation
    B. Cardiac arrhythmias
    C. Ascites
    D. Increased intracranial pressures

28. Following knee surgery, a patient has a sequential compression device (SCD). The nurse should:

    A. Change SCD settings according to patient comfort
    B. Discontinue the SCD during patient ambulation
    C. Keep the SCD in place when removing initial dressing
    D. Elevate the SCD on two pillows

29. Your male patient, who has a diagnosis of chronic liver failure, has deficient vitamin K absorption. Which assessment findings indicate vitamin K deficiency?

    A. Testicular atrophy and gynecomastia
    B. Petechiae and ecchymosis
    C. Ascites and orthopnea
    D. Dyspnea and fatigue

30. The physician has ordered several laboratory tests to help diagnose an infant's bleeding disorder. Which of the following tests, if abnormal, would the nurse interpret as most likely to indicate hemophilia?

   A. Reticulocyte count
   B. Fibrin degradation products (FDP)
   C. Bleeding time
   D. Activated partial thromboplastin time (APTT)

31. Of the following, follicle-stimulating hormone (FSH) is primarily responsible for:

   A. Maintaining the corpus luteum
   B. Spermatogenesis
   C. Testosterone production
   D. Stimulating ovulation

32. Which of the following is not a type of cardiomyopathy?

   A. Constrictive
   B. Restrictive
   C. Hypertrophic
   D. Dilated

33. You are assigned to care for Mr. O., a 65-year-old male, recently admitted to the hospital with a diagnosis of left-sided congestive heart-failure. In your assessment, you should expect to find:

   A. Crushing chest pain
   B. Dyspnea on exertion
   C. Jugular vein distention
   D. Extensive peripheral edema

34. You are caring for a patient who has a tumor affecting the anterior pituitary gland. Secretion of which of the following hormones is least likely to be affected?

    A. Prolactin
    B. Oxytocin
    C. Thyroid-stimulating hormone
    D. Luteinizing hormone

35. You are caring for a patient who experienced a spinal injury and is now paraplegic. You understand that the highest vertebra in which a fracture affecting the spinal column can occur while still only causing paraplegia instead of quadriplegia is which of the following?

    A. T1
    B. T2
    C. T6
    D. C7

36. Which of the following statements made by a patient with amyotrophic lateral sclerosis (ALS) is correct?

    A. "I will have periods of remission and periods of exacerbation."
    B. "I will gradually become completely paralyzed."
    C. "Only a very small percentage of people with ALS survive."
    D. "The progression of ALS can be stopped by using steroids."

37. You are caring for a patient who has a gastrostomy tube. You are preparing to give your patient his morning medications through the tube. What preventative measure is necessary to avoid tube obstruction?

    A. Monitor for GI distention
    B. Assess for GI distress
    C. Keep head of bed elevated 30-45 degrees during feedings
    D. Flush the tube with 30 mL of warm water before and after medication administration

38. You are assessing a patient who has a pressure ulcer over the sacrum that is 2 mm deep, 4 cm wide, and 3 cm long with subcutaneous tissues visible in the top half and black eschar in the bottom half. What is the best way to describe this pressure ulcer?

    A. Stage IV
    B. Unstageable
    C. Deep tissue injury
    D. Stage III

39. During this phase of the menstrual cycle, the endometrial thickness increases six-fold due to a spike in estrogen levels, and the cervical mucus changes to become more favorable to sperm:

    A. Ischemic phase
    B. Menstrual phase
    C. Proliferative phase
    D. Secretory phase

40. If ischemia is severe or lasts too long, it can cause a heart attack (myocardial infarction) and can lead to heart tissue death. In most cases, a temporary blood shortage to the heart causes chest pain. But, in other cases, there is no pain. These cases are called *silent ischemia*. Of the following, the patient most at risk for silent ischemia is:

    A. A patient with coronary artery disease and chronic pancreatitis
    B. A patient with coronary artery disease who has just started to exercise
    C. A patient with coronary artery disease and Cushing's disease
    D. A patient with coronary artery disease and diabetes mellitus

41. You are caring for a patient with cystic fibrosis who asks you what the chances are that their children will have this condition. Which response is appropriate?

    A. "Only people with cystic fibrosis will have children who are carriers for the disease."
    B. "Pulmonary fibrosis, not cystic fibrosis, is a genetic disease."

C. "Cystic fibrosis is a genetic condition. I can refer you to a genetic counselor."

D. "Genetics plays a small role in the transmission of cystic fibrosis, but there are other factors to consider."

42. Propylthiouracil (PTU) is a medication that inhibits the synthesis of:

A. Adrenocorticotropic hormone (ACTH)
B. Glucagon
C. Thyroid hormones
D. Parathyroid hormone (PTH)

43. All of the following statements related to scoliosis are true except:

A. A majority of scoliosis cases are of idiopathic etiology
B. Leg length discrepancy can cause functional scoliosis
C. Congenital scoliosis results from malformation of vertebral structures
D. Scoliosis is the lateral curvature that only occurs in the thoracic spine

44. The most common bariatric surgical procedure is:

A. Biliopancreatic Diversion with Duodenal Switch Gastric Bypass (BPD/DS)
B. Roux-en-Y Gastric Bypass (RYGB)
C. Sleeve Gastrectomy
D. Adjustable Gastric Band (AGB)

45. Erythropoietin is produced by the:

A. Adrenal gland
B. Pituitary gland
C. Kidneys
D. Thalamus

46. When a patient has an elevated blood urea nitrogen (BUN), the nurse understands that all of the following factors can elevate this level except:

A. GI bleeding
B. Dehydration
C. Poor renal perfusion
D. Diabetes mellitus

47. Which of the following individuals is most at risk for coronary artery disease (CAD)?

A. A pre-menopausal, obese Caucasian female who has never smoked
B. A post-menopausal, Asian woman with diabetes who is not a current smoker
C. A Native American, obese male who has never smoked
D. An African American male with hypertension and a positive family history of CAD

48. Which of the following tests allows for best visualization of the bronchi?

A. Chest MRI
B. Bronchoscopy
C. Chest CT scan
D. Chest X-ray

49. You are caring for a patient who just underwent a thyroidectomy. For the first 72 hours, you would assess your patient for Chvostek's sign because it would indicate:

A. Hyponatremia
B. Hypocalcemia
C. Hypermagnesemia
D. Hypokalemia

50. Straightening of a joint that increases the angle between two articulating bones is:

   A. Flexion
   B. Abduction
   C. Adduction
   D. Extension

51. Which of the following medications is an antibiotic commonly used in inflammatory bowel disease to treat or prevent infections related to the loss of normal flora in the gut?

   A. Cyclosporine (Neoral, Restasis)
   B. Prednisone (Deltasone)
   C. 5-ASA (Pentasa, Asacol)
   D. Metronidazole (Flagyl)

52. You are caring for an 82-year-old male patient admitted to the hospital the previous day with COPD exacerbation. Since admission, he has not eaten well and refuses to get out of bed because he can't "catch his breath."

During your assessment, you notice a 2-cm red spot with localized warmth located over the sacrum that is blanchable. How should this area be documented?

   A. Deep tissue injury
   B. Stage I pressure ulcer
   C. Erythema
   D. Hematoma

53. Which of the following is not a risk factor for bladder cancer?

   A. Working in a factory that manufactures rubber parts
   B. Smoking
   C. Heavy alcohol use
   D. History of radiation to the pelvic area

54. Which of the following is true about cardiac tamponade?

    A. Cardiac tamponade is a procedure done to stop bleeding from coronary arteries
    B. Cardiac tamponade is a condition that occurs when fluid builds up around the heart
    C. Cardiac tamponade is a percussive test used to understand the function of the cardiac valves
    D. Cardiac tamponade refers to a tool used to soak blood from around the heart during cardiothoracic surgery

55. Which of the following statements is true related to pulmonary tuberculosis?

    A. Active pulmonary tuberculosis is diagnosed by a chest x-ray
    B. An intradermal tuberculin skin test (PPD) reading of 6 mm is negative for a person who is immunosuppressed
    C. Tuberculosis is primarily spread by droplets
    D. People who have been vaccinated with the bacille Calmette-Guerin (BCG) vaccine will have a positive response to an intradermal tuberculin purified protein derivative (PPD) skin test

56. What is the most common complication that occurs in insulin-treated patients?

    A. Hypoglycemia
    B. Peripheral neuropathy
    C. Kidney disease
    D. Diabetic ketoacidosis (DKA)

57. How many pairs of ribs attach directly to the sternum?

    A. Twelve
    B. Five
    C. Eight
    D. Seven

58. You are providing teaching to a patient with ulcerative colitis. Which of the following statements indicates the need for further teaching?

A. "Ulcerative colitis can cause bleeding in my intestines."
B. "Ulcerative colitis can appear anywhere in my intestines."
C. "Ulcerative colitis is not associated with race, gender, or social class."
D. "Ulcerative colitis will make it harder for me to absorb nutrients."

59. Which of the following disorders results from a deficiency of factor VIII?

A. Hemophilia
B. Christmas disease
C. Sickle cell disease
D. Disseminated intravascular coagulation (DIC)

60. Which of the following statements related to serum creatinine levels in the diagnosis of renal failure is true?

A. It does not provide any information about muscle metabolism or indicate renal failure
B. It measures the end product of muscle metabolism and is an excellent indicator of renal failure
C. It does not provide any information about muscle metabolism but is an excellent indicator of renal failure
D. It measures the end product of muscle metabolism but does not indicate renal failure

61. What are the most common symptoms of digoxin toxicity?

A. Abdominal pain & altered mental status
B. Arrhythmias & chest pain
C. Abdominal pain & arrhythmias
D. Nausea & vomiting

62. You are reviewing your patient's arterial blood gas (ABG) values, and you note the following:

    - pH 7.36
    - PCO2 55 mm Hg
    - HCO3 27 mEq/L

    What do you interpret these values as?

    A. Compensated respiratory alkalosis
    B. Compensated respiratory acidosis
    C. Uncompensated respiratory alkalosis
    D. Uncompensated respiratory acidosis

63. Which of the following conditions is caused by long-term exposure to high levels of cortisol?

    A. Addison's disease
    B. Adrenal insufficiency
    C. Hyperpituitarism
    D. Cushing's syndrome

64. Which of the following fractures is least likely to cause a fat embolism?

    A. Humerus fracture
    B. Rib fracture
    C. Radius fracture
    D. Pelvic fracture

65. What is an indication for initiating enteral feedings?

    A. Paralytic ileus
    B. Inadequate intake for the previous 3 to 5 days
    C. GI bleeding and/or ischemia
    D. Intractable vomiting

66. Which of the following, also called the "tissue factor," is part of the extrinsic coagulation pathway, and is also known as Factor III?

    A. Proconvertin
    B. Fibrinogen
    C. Prothrombin
    D. Thromboplastin

67. The nurse is teaching a patient with interstitial cystitis about her condition. The nurse is aware:

    A. Bladder capacity is reduced in this condition due to obstruction
    B. The patient will need to be on daily aspirin therapy
    C. The patient's cystoscopy may reveal bladder hemorrhage
    D. Up to 95% of all cases occur in young men

68. You are providing your patient with discharge education about warfarin (Coumadin), which was initiated during his hospitalization after a cardiac valve replacement. During your teaching, you explain the potential interactions of warfarin with certain medications. All of the following medications may potentiate warfarin except:

    A. Acetaminophen (Tylenol)
    B. Steroids
    C. Aspirin
    D. Glucagons

69. You are receiving shift report. Which of the following patients should you see first?

    A. A patient admitted with viral meningitis who needs to receive IV antibiotics
    B. A patient admitted for asthma exacerbation complaining of shortness of breath after using a bronchodilator inhaler
    C. A client with chronic obstructive pulmonary disease who has a pulse oximetry reading of 91% and clubbing fingers

D. A patient with possible C-diff who needs a stool specimen sent to laboratory

70. Which of the following statements is true related to antidiuretic hormone (ADH)?

   A. It is stored in the anterior pituitary gland
   B. It is synthesized by the posterior pituitary gland
   C. It is stored in the hypothalamus
   D. It is synthesized in the hypothalamus

71. You are assessing your patient's adaptation to the changes in functional status after a cerebrovascular accident (stroke). You determine that the patient is most successfully adapting if she:

   A. Experiences bouts of depression and irritability
   B. Refuses to use modified feeding utensils
   C. Gets angry with family if they interrupt a task
   D. Consistently uses assistive devices when dressing herself

72. You are supervising a student nurse who is caring for a 43-year-old male who has chronic pancreatitis. Which of the following statements made by the student to the patient indicates that they need more teaching?

   A. "Chronic pancreatitis tends to have periods of remission and periods of exacerbation."
   B. "Avoiding alcohol is recommended."
   C. "Most people who have chronic pancreatitis do not die because of it."
   D. "The cause of chronic pancreatitis is alcohol abuse."

73. Which of the following statements is true related to first degree burns?

   A. They will likely lead to permanent scarring
   B. They do not extend into the epidermis
   C. They may develop into second degree burns as the inflammatory response develops
   D. They never blister

74. Gross, painless hematuria is commonly the first symptom of:

    A. Polycystic kidney disease (PKD)
    B. Kidney stones
    C. Bladder cancer
    D. Nephrotic syndrome

75. Baroreceptors monitor blood pressure and help us to respond to shock. These are found in the:

    A. Carotid arteries and aortic arch
    B. Abdominal aorta
    C. Brain and spinal cord
    D. Brain and ventricular muscle tissue

76. Chronic bronchitis is characterized by which of the following clinical manifestations?

    A. Respiratory alkalosis
    B. Chronic non-productive cough
    C. Pulmonary hypertension in the late stages
    D. Left-sided heart failure in the late stages

77. A low thyroid-stimulating hormone (TSH) level with elevated triiodothyronine (T3) and thyroxine (T4) levels indicates:

    A. Secondary hyperthyroidism
    B. Secondary hypothyroidism
    C. Primary hyperparathyroidism
    D. Primary hyperthyroidism

78. Possible complications following total joint (TJA) surgery include all of the following except:

    A. Pulmonary embolism
    B. Deep vein thrombosis
    C. Compartment syndrome

D. Impaired bladder function

79. All of the following statements related to enteral nutrition are true except:

A. It is associated with fewer complications than parenteral nutrition
B. It maintains gastrointestinal structure and function by maintaining villi height and number and enzyme activity
C. It is indicated for complete intestinal obstruction
D. It maintains the mucosal barrier of the GI tract

80. A female client is brought to the emergency department with deep partial-thickness and full-thickness (second- and third-degree) burns on the left arm, left leg, and anterior trunk. Using the rule of nines, what is the total body surface area that has been burned?

A. 54%
B. 27%
C. 36%
D. 45%

81. A patient is scheduled for an intravenous pyelogram. The priority nursing action before the test would be to:

A. Determine if there is a patient history of iodine or seafood allergy
B. Administer radiopaque dye
C. Administer a sedative
D. Ensure the patient is NPO

82. Mean arterial pressure (MAP) is calculated by using which of the following formulas?

A. [(2 x DBP)+SBP] / 3
B. [(3 x DBP)+SBP] / 2
C. [(2 x SBP)+DBP] / 3
D. [(3 x SBP)+DBP] / 2

83. The most common respiratory cause of death in the United States is:

    A. Pneumonia
    B. Pulmonary embolism
    C. Chronic obstructive pulmonary disease (COPD)
    D. Status asthmaticus

84. This acts as a brace to hold the arm away from the thorax:

    A. Sternoclavicular joint
    B. Xiphoid process
    C. Clavicle
    D. Scapula

85. You are completing discharge instructions with a patient who has been treated for hepatitis A. In your discharge teaching, you should include all of the following except:

    A. The patient is at high risk for developing hepatic cancer
    B. Compliance with the treatment plan is necessary to prevent exacerbations; relapse can and does occasionally occur
    C. Hepatitis A usually resolves with no residual problems
    D. The patient should never donate blood

86. According to the National Pressure Ulcer Advisory Panel (NPUAP), an intact, serum-filled blister is classified as which of the following?

    A. A suspected deep tissue injury
    B. A stage II pressure ulcer
    C. An unstageable pressure ulcer
    D. A stage I pressure ulcer

87. A female patient is being treated for genital herpes. She should be educated about the:

    A. Need to keep the perineal area moist
    B. Need to wear tight-fitting nylon underwear

C. Prevention of outbreaks and lesions

D. Need to abstain from sexual intercourse while lesions are present

88. Cardiomyopathy is a cardiac disease involving which of the following?

A. Myocardium

B. Left anterior descending coronary artery

C. Aorta

D. Chordae tendineae

89. A patient admitted to the medical-surgical floor with pneumonia is receiving supplemental oxygen at 2 L/minute via nasal cannula. The patient's history includes chronic obstructive pulmonary disease (COPD) and coronary artery disease (CAD). Because of these history findings, the nurse closely monitors the oxygen flow and the patient's respiratory status.

Which of the following complications may arise if the patient receives a high oxygen concentration?

A. Apnea

B. Respiratory alkalosis

C. Anginal pain

D. Metabolic acidosis

90. Thyroid-stimulating hormone (TSH) is secreted by the:

A. Adrenal glands

B. Hypothalamus

C. Anterior pituitary gland

D. Posterior pituitary gland

91. Which of the following is not a potential complication of myasthenia gravis?

A. Cholinergic crisis

B. Aspiration pneumonia

C. Starvation

D. Myasthenia crisis

92. The most common presenting symptoms in patients with disorders of the gastrointestinal tract include:

    A. Nausea/vomiting, evidence of bleeding, weight loss
    B. Evidence of bleeding, pain, nausea/vomiting
    C. Pain, nausea/vomiting, change in bowel pattern
    D. Pain, change in bowel pattern, evidence of bleeding

93. Which of the following serve as the first line of defense against microorganisms, acting as phagocytes?

    A. Basophils
    B. Neutrophils
    C. Granulocytes
    D. Eosinophils

94. Which of the following statements is true related to renal hormones?

    A. Renin is released from the kidneys in response to hypoperfusion
    B. Erythropoietin stimulates bone marrow production of ferritin
    C. Prostaglandins are primarily produced in the renal cortex
    D. Vitamin D is necessary for absorption of phosphorus through the gastrointestinal tract

95. Which of the following findings in a patient awaiting abdominal aneurysm repair would you report immediately to the physician?

    A. Severe back pain
    B. Increased fatigue
    C. Increased cyanosis of the feet
    D. Swelling of the arms and face

96. Which of the following statements is true related to laryngeal cancer?

    A. Tumors of the subglottis are the most common form of laryngeal cancer

B. Race is not a risk factor for the development of this disease, but it is more likely to occur in women

C. Tumors that develop from squamous cells are the largest cause of malignant laryngeal cancer

D. Diagnosis of laryngeal cancer is by CT scan

97. All of the following are signs and symptoms associated with diabetic ketoacidosis (DKA) except:

   A. Hyperglycemia
   B. Metabolic alkalosis
   C. Dehydration
   D. Polyuria

98. You are caring for a patient who has a tonic-clonic seizure. Which of the following interventions is most important during the seizure?

   A. Hold the patient down so they do not injure themselves
   B. Protect the patient's airway by using a tongue blade or intubating if possible
   C. Check the patient's blood glucose level
   D. Ensure the patient's environment is safe

99. The physician has ordered a paracentesis for a patient with ascites. Prior to the procedure, the nurse:

   A. Keeps the patient NPO for 24 hours
   B. Instructs the patient to void
   C. Administers laxatives and a soap suds enema
   D. Prepares the patient for transfer to the operating room

100. A hospital employee is given a tuberculin skin test. When the nurse reads the test 48 hours after administration, it is positive. This is an example of which of the following types of hypersensitivity reactions?

   A. Type II cytotoxic hypersensitivity reaction
   B. Type I immediate hypersensitivity reaction

C. Type IV cell-mediated hypersensitivity reaction

D. Type III immune complex hypersensitivity reaction

101. Which of the following patients would not be a candidate for an urinary catheter?

    A. A 87-year-old female with sepsis whose urinary output was 40 mL over the last four hours

    B. A 30-year-old male who is not able void voluntarily but who needs to provide a urine specimen for a diagnostic decision

    C. A 43-year-old female who had a pelvic fracture from an MVA and needs monitoring of her kidney function

    D. A 53-year-old male who has been unable to void for 12 hours and has bladder distention

102. Which of the following statements is true related to an apical pulse?

    A. It is palpated on the side of the neck

    B. It is auscultated over the heart with a stethoscope

    C. It is palpated at the wrist

    D. It is auscultated on the top of the foot with a Doppler

103. Which of the following is not a risk factor for developing a spontaneous pneumothorax?

    A. Smoking

    B. High-altitude flying

    C. Being a young male who is tall and slender

    D. Combat in the armed forces

104. The most common cause of death in people with cystic fibrosis (CF) is:

    A. Respiratory failure

    B. Lung cancer

    C. Opportunistic infection

    D. Dehydration

105. What disease of the musculoskeletal system is considered an autoimmune disorder?

    A. Osteoporosis
    B. Scoliosis
    C. Rheumatoid arthritis
    D. Osteoarthritis

106. Which of the following complications is not associated with peptic ulcer disease (PUD)?

    A. Hyperemesis gravidarum
    B. Perforation
    C. Obstruction of the pyloric area
    D. GI hemorrhage

107. The nurse would instruct the patient with pernicious anemia to eat which of the following foods to obtain the best supply of vitamin B12?

    A. Meats and dairy products
    B. Citrus fruits
    C. Whole grains
    D. Green leafy vegetables

108. Which of the following is most likely to be the first symptom noticed by someone who has bladder cancer?

    A. Pain in the low abdomen
    B. A patient with bladder cancer will not have symptoms
    C. Blood in the urine
    D. Frequent urination

109. About how many deaths in the United States annually are the result of cardiovascular disease?

    A. 230,000
    B. 1,150,000

C. 900,000

D. 600,000

110. You are caring for a patient with COPD. Her ABG shows the following:

- PaO_2 180
- pH 7.36
- CO_2 49
- HCO_3 32

Which of the following interventions should you consider?

A. Prepare to administer sodium bicarbonate

B. Administer a nebulized bronchodilator

C. Decrease the amount of oxygen being given to the patient

D. Begin providing the patient with bag valve mask respirations

111. Which of the following statements is true related to metformin (Glucophage)?

A. It delays the absorption of carbohydrates in the intestine by slowing gastric emptying

B. It causes hypersecretion of insulin

C. It increases insulin sensitivity

D. It decreases hepatic glucose production by increasing hepatic glycogenolysis

112. Which of the following best describes decorticate posturing?

A. The body is lying facing upward with the palms of the hands open and facing upward

B. The arms are bent inward, fists are clenched, and the legs are held out straight

C. The legs are bent at the knees when the neck is flexed so that the chin touches the chest

D. The arms are held out straight and turned outward, the fists are clenched, and the legs are held out straight

113. You are caring for a 34-year-old male with acute appendicitis who is scheduled for surgery the following day. He starts complaining of increasing abdominal pain. Vital signs are BP 86/52, HR 114, RR 24, Temp 101.5, O2 sat 100% on room air. You note on your assessment that the patient's abdomen is tender and rigid, and the patient is diaphoretic. Which of the following interventions is least important for this patient?

    A. Administer IV fluids
    B. Administer IV antibiotics
    C. Prepare for an earlier surgery
    D. Perform an abdominal CT

114. Which skin condition is of the greatest concern for someone with type one diabetes mellitus?

    A. Diabetic ulcers
    B. Diabetic neuropathy
    C. Osteomyelitis
    D. Chronic dryness

115. You are caring for a patient with chronic kidney disease (CKD) and his recent lab work reveals he has a serum potassium level of 6.8 mEq/L. What should you assess first?

    A. Respirations
    B. Blood pressure
    C. Pulse
    D. Temperature

116. Electrical activity of the heart is facilitated by the transmembranal exchange of all of the following ions except:

    A. Potassium
    B. Sodium
    C. Calcium
    D. Phosphorous

117. All of the following statements related to the lower airway are true except:

    A. Cells in the alveolar walls secrete surfactant
    B. The right bronchus is slightly wider and shorter than the left
    C. The alveoli are surrounded by pulmonary capillaries
    D. The terminal bronchioles are partially surrounded by cartilage to resist collapse

118. The nurse understands that which of the following is true about a pheochromocytoma?

    A. A pheochromocytoma can cause hypertension
    B. A pheochromocytoma is a type of tumor that releases adrenocorticotropic hormone (ACTH)
    C. A pheochromocytoma that is big enough should be palpated during assessment to accurately determine its size
    D. A pheochromocytoma is type of benign skin lesion that is often found in patients with liver disease

119. The most common diagnostic study used to assess the musculoskeletal system and monitor effects of treatment is:

    A. Magnetic resonance imaging (MRI)
    B. X-ray
    C. Computed tomography (CT) scan
    D. Bone scan

120. You are performing preoperative teaching with a patient who has ulcerative colitis (UC) and needs a total colectomy with an ileoanal reservoir. Which information do you include?

    A. The surgery usually occurs in two stages
    B. A reservoir is created that exits through the abdominal wall
    C. Continence is not possible after this surgery
    D. A permanent ileostomy is created

121. Your patient is suspected to have liver failure and is getting diagnostic testing done to confirm this diagnosis. Which electrolyte imbalance is most commonly seen in liver failure?

    A. Hyperkalemia
    B. Hypomagnesemia
    C. Hypermagnesemia
    D. Hypokalemia

122. You are caring for a patient who has multiple myeloma. You understand that this cancer is primarily located in which of the following?

    A. Hematopoietic stem cells
    B. Osteoblasts
    C. Bone marrow
    D. Lymph nodes

123. All of the following statements related to a transurethral resection of the prostate (TURP) are true except:

    A. Complications may include bleeding and urethral stricture
    B. TURP requires longer recovery times
    C. TURP must be performed when a patient is diagnosed with benign prostatic hyperplasia (BPH)
    D. Flow rates with this procedure appear to be better than any other therapy

124. The exchange of gases and nutrients between blood and tissues is a major function of:

    A. Arteries
    B. Arterioles
    C. Capillaries
    D. Veins

125. When reviewing the chart of your patient with long-standing chronic obstructive pulmonary disease (COPD), you should pay close attention to the results of which pulmonary function test?

    A. Residual volume
    B. Functional residual capacity
    C. Total lung capacity
    D. FEV1/FVC ratio

126. Treatment of hyperosmolar hyperglycemic syndrome (HHS) includes all of the following except:

    A. Fluids to correct severe dehydration
    B. Correction of electrolyte imbalances
    C. Metformin to treat the hyperglycemia
    D. Treatment of any underlying disease

127. You are caring for a patient who has chronic osteomyelitis. Which statement made by the patient indicates that further teaching is needed?

    A. "Treating this kind of infection is very difficult."
    B. "People with osteomyelitis are at a much higher risk of needing an amputation."
    C. "This kind of infection often requires surgery."
    D. "I will need to take antibiotic pills for at least a week to get rid of this infection."

128. Which of the following is not given to treat anemia?

    A. Iron
    B. Vitamin B12 (cobalamin)
    C. Vitamin B3 (niacin)
    D. Vitamin B9 (folate)

129. A patient tells you that he is concerned about getting polycystic kidney disease (PKD). Which of the following questions should you ask to better understand his risk for this disease?

    A. "Have you had kidney stones before?"
    B. "Do you drink two or more alcohol beverages each day?"
    C. "Do you have any history of injuries to your kidney area?"
    D. "Has anyone in your family ever had PKD?"

130. Which of the following is true about mean arterial pressure (MAP)?

    A. Any MAP over 70 is healthy
    B. A patient's MAP may sometimes exceed their systolic blood pressure
    C. MAP is average blood pressure in the arteries
    D. MAP is calculated by taking the average of the systolic and diastolic blood pressures

131. A nurse is caring for an elderly patient with congestive heart failure. The nurse keeps in mind that respiratory changes associated with aging include diminished effectiveness of gas exchange between alveolus and capillary walls leading to:

    A. An increase in pH and pCO_2
    B. Thinning of pulmonary vasculature
    C. A decline in pO_2 and O_2 saturation
    D. Thinning of moist mucous membranes

132. You are treating a patient who has diabetic ketoacidosis (DKA) and are administering regular insulin IV. Which of the follow laboratory values is most important to monitor during your treatment of this patient?

    A. Potassium
    B. Troponin
    C. Creatinine
    D. Magnesium

133. While assessing a male patient, the nurse asks him to rotate his head forcibly against resistance applied to the side of his chin. The nurse then asks him to shrug his shoulders against resistance.

Which of the following cranial nerves is the nurse assessing?

   A. VII (Facial)
   B. XI (Accessory)
   C. XII (Hypoglossal)
   D. V (Trigeminal)

134. Your patient, Mr. S., was admitted to the medical-surgical unit for a gastrointestinal bleed associated with a duodenal ulcer. You are completing an admission assessment on him. Which of the following statements do you know is true related to clinical manifestations of gastrointestinal bleeding?

   A. Platelet counts initially decrease due to delayed coagulation process
   B. Massive blood loss leads to venous, then peripheral artery dilation
   C. Vasomotor instability is the most sensitive indicator of blood loss
   D. Dark, tarry stools indicate rapid blood loss

135. Which of the following is not a likely cause of disseminated intravascular coagulation (DIC)?

   A. Hemolytic transfusion reaction
   B. Transplant rejection
   C. Preterm labor
   D. Septicemia

136. A patient is admitted with chronic pyelonephritis. The nurse is aware:

   A. White blood cells will be absent on this patient's urinalysis, with heavy growth of bacteria
   B. Hypertension is a late symptom of the disease
   C. The condition often results from chronic obstruction of the urinary tract
   D. Flank pain is likely to be extremely severe in this condition

137. Your patient with a diagnosis of congestive heart failure is scheduled for cardiac catheterization. You are aware that:

   A. The patient is at increased risk for fluid overload due to the osmotic effect of the contrast agent
   B. You will need to watch for osmotic diuresis, which can result in hypertension
   C. Following the procedure, the patient must be kept in bed with no bending of the extremity that was used for the catheterization for 8 hours
   D. The patient will not be able to eat or drink for 4 hours before the procedure

138. The most common cause of transudative pleural effusion is:

   A. Liver failure
   B. Infection
   C. Cancer
   D. Congestive heart failure

139. For which of the following patients would a hemoglobin A1C not provide usable information?

   A. A 65-year-old male with heart failure who had 80 mg of furosemide (Lasix) over the last 12 hours
   B. A 23-year-old male with type one diabetes mellitus who had a splenectomy two years ago
   C. A 13-year-old female who has type one diabetes mellitus and spina bifida
   D. A 32-year-old female with gestational diabetes who has just been diagnosed with preeclampsia

140. Which of the following symptoms would be least likely to occur in someone who has multiple sclerosis?

   A. Seizures
   B. Visual disturbances
   C. Bowel dysfunction

D. Depression

141. A patient with acute pancreatitis is to be started on parenteral nutrition. Contraindications for parenteral nutrition include all of the following except:

   A. Complete intestinal obstruction
   B. Health care directives that decline parenteral nutrition
   C. A functional gastrointestinal tract
   D. No venous access

142. You are caring for an immobilized patient, and after thorough assessment, you chart that a pressure ulcer is present on the patient's sacrum with visible subcutaneous fat and slough that does not obscure the base of the wound.

What stage pressure ulcer would this be classified as, based on the description?

   A. Stage II
   B. Stage IV
   C. Unstageable
   D. Stage III

143. Which of the following statements regarding urine specific gravity determination is false?

   A. Normal is 1.010 to 1.025
   B. The dipstick method is the most common method of measuring specific gravity
   C. Increase in specific gravity indicates urine that is more highly concentrated than normal
   D. Increase in specific gravity indicates increased renal perfusion

144. What is the most comprehensive and most accurate way to diagnose myocardial infarction?

   A. Patient reports of chest pain

B. Angiography

C. EKG changes

D. Elevated troponin

145. You are caring for a patient who is sensitive to the opioid pain medications you have administered and develops bradypnea with an O2 sat that dips to 85%. Which of the following would you expect to see on the patient's ABG?

A. Compensated respiratory alkalosis

B. Compensated respiratory acidosis

C. Uncompensated respiratory alkalosis

D. Uncompensated respiratory acidosis

146. A patient has just been started on tolbutamide (Orinase). Which of the following statements does the nurse know to be true about this medication?

A. This medication is preferred over other oral sulfonylureas as it only needs to be given once daily

B. Starting daily dose is usually 250 mg daily

C. Duration of action is 6-12 hours

D. It is cleared through the feces

147. A patient with osteoarthritis (OA) states that her friend with rheumatoid arthritis (RA) takes steroid pills for his condition, and asks why she is not prescribed these same pills. Which of the following would be the best explanation by the nurse?

A. Oral corticosteroids can be used for osteoarthritis (OA)

B. Osteoarthritis (OA) and rheumatoid arthritis (RA) are similar conditions

C. Intra-articular corticosteroid injections are used to treat osteoarthritis (OA)

D. Osteoarthritis (OA) is treated using systemic treatment routes

148. Which of the following dietary considerations is true for a patient who is diagnosed with a volvulus?

    A. The patient can only have clear fluids
    B. The patient should be made NPO
    C. The patient should follow a high-fiber, high-protein diet
    D. The patient may have a full fluid diet except for milk

149. You are assessing a patient who has three areas of pressure-related skin breakdown over the sacral region that are close together. Tunneling connects two of these areas. What is the best way to document your skin assessment?

    A. Document this as one pressure ulcer with areas of intact skin
    B. Document these as three pressure ulcers, and note the tunneling when documenting both of the ulcers to which the tunneling is connected
    C. Document the isolated pressure ulcer as one pressure ulcer, and the two that are connected with tunneling as one pressure ulcer
    D. Document these as three pressure ulcers, and note the tunneling when documenting the ulcer that the tunneling appears to have originated from

150. The outermost layer of the kidney is referred to as the:

    A. Hilum
    B. Medulla
    C. Renal pelvis
    D. Cortex

Answer Key

Q.	1	2	3	4	5	6	7	8	9	10	11	12	13	14	15
A.	C	D	C	D	C	B	A	D	A	B	D	B	A	B	D

Q.	16	17	18	19	20	21	22	23	24	25	26	27	28	29	30
A.	D	A	B	C	D	D	C	D	D	A	B	B	B	B	D

Q.	31	32	33	34	35	36	37	38	39	40	41	42	43	44	45
A.	B	A	B	B	A	B	D	B	C	D	C	C	D	B	C

Q.	46	47	48	49	50	51	52	53	54	55	56	57	58	59	60
A.	D	D	B	B	D	D	C	C	B	D	A	D	B	A	D

Q.	61	62	63	64	65	66	67	68	69	70	71	72	73	74	75
A.	D	B	D	B	B	D	C	A	B	D	D	D	D	C	A

Q.	76	77	78	79	80	81	82	83	84	85	86	87	88	89	90
A.	C	D	D	C	D	A	A	C	C	A	B	D	A	A	C

Q.	91	92	93	94	95	96	97	98	99	100	101	102	103	104	105
A.	C	C	B	A	A	C	B	D	B	C	C	B	D	A	C

Q.	106	107	108	109	110	111	112	113	114	115	116	117	118	119	120
A.	A	A	C	D	C	C	B	D	A	C	D	D	A	B	A

Q.	121	122	123	124	125	126	127	128	129	130	131	132	133	134	135
A.	D	C	C	C	D	C	D	C	C	D	C	A	B	C	C

Q.	136	137	138	139	140	141	142	143	144	145	146	147	148	149	150
A.	C	D	D	B	A	A	D	D	B	D	D	C	C	B	D

Answers and Explanations

1. C - An oral cholecystogram, or GB series, is an x-ray exam to visualize the gallbladder by administering, by mouth, a radiopaque contrast agent that is excreted by the liver. The patient is to be NPO after administration of the oral dye (cannot eat or drink anything).

2. D - Intrinsic factor (IF) is required for the absorption of vitamin B12.

3. C - The vas deferens is a duct that transports sperm from the epididymis (structure that curves over testes) to the urethra.

4. D - Acute renal failure is often reversible and can be recovered from without long-term kidney damage in many situations.

5. C - Obstructive shock is associated with physical obstruction of the great vessels or the heart itself, resulting in an inability of the heart to fill or to eject blood effectively. Increased pressure in the thoracic cavity or tension pneumothorax is common with this type of shock, preventing blood return from the head to the thoracic cavity, resulting in distended neck veins.

6. B - The pleura is a double-layered membrane that covers the lung and inside of the thorax. The parietal pleural membrane lines the inside of the thoracic cavity, while the visceral pleural membrane lines the surface of the lungs.

7. A - Levemir is a *long-acting* insulin, not a rapid-acting insulin. Rapid-acting insulins include Humalog, Novolog, and Apidra.

8. D - Patients with rheumatoid arthritis (RA), including those in the early stages, often experience early morning stiffness in their joints that typically lasts more than one hour.

9. A - The advantage of this procedure, also called the TIPS procedure, is that it can be performed in the interventional radiology department; it is a minimally invasive procedure by which stents connect portal and

hepatic veins under radiographic guidance. This decreases pressure in the portal vein and subsequently on the varices to prevent rupture and bleeding.

10. B - A negative test result indicates that no HIV antibodies were detected in the blood sample. However, if initial HIV screening tests are negative, they should be repeated in 3 months to detect any infections that had not yet led to seroconversion. The other options are incorrect.

11. D - Cardiac is calculated by multiplying stroke volume by heart rate. A healthy heart with a normal cardiac output pumps 4 to 8 liters of blood every minute.

12. B - Broad spectrum antibiotics are started initially until an organism is identified on a culture specimen, and the antibiotic is changed to one to which the organism is sensitive.

13. A - The patient is having a hypoglycemic episode. Because the patient is still conscious with an intact swallowing response, the 15/15 rule is generally applied; administer 15 grams of a fast-acting carbohydrate and wait 15 minutes. Repeat as needed, until blood glucose levels are greater than 70 mg/dL.

14. B - The motor and postural changes that Parkinson's disease creates often leads to joint or muscle pain. This is a common complication of this disease.

15. D - Peptic ulcer disease is caused by lifestyle choices, genetic factors, and *H. pylori* infections. NSAID use, smoking, and stress are all factors that increase the risk of PUD.

16. D - Basal cell carcinoma in an invasive epidermal tumor with a low rate of metastasis.

17. A - The accuracy of a urine pregnancy test is greatest 6 weeks after last menstrual period.

18. B - Routes for administering nitroglycerine in treating cardiac ischemia include sublingually, intravenously, topically, and orally.

19. C - The lower airway consists of the bronchial airway and lungs. The structure of the two mainstream bronchi resembles the trachea. Five lobar bronchi diverge from the two mainstream bronchi to enter the lobes of the lungs. The lobar bronchi further divide into progressively smaller airways called terminal bronchioles. Alveoli are the air sacs of the respiratory system where oxygen and carbon dioxide exchange takes place.

20. D - Addison's disease is a chronic endocrine system disorder in which the adrenal glands do not produce sufficient steroid hormones (glucocorticoids and mineralocorticoids); it involves the destruction of the adrenal cortex, resulting in adrenocortical hypofunction.

21. D - An immovable joint in which bones come into direct contact with each other is known as synarthrosis. The bones are separated only by a thin layer of fibrous connective tissue; cranial suture joints are an example.

22. C - Esophageal varices are *not* a complication of GERD, but rather a complication of liver failure (most often a consequence of portal hypertension, commonly due to cirrhosis).

23. D - Mast cells are body, not blood, cells; they are a type of polymorphonuclear leukocyte located in the skin just outside of the capillaries. Mast cells play a prominent role in the activation of the allergy response. When a person has an allergy, mast cells respond to harmless triggers as if they were a threat.

24. D - Pyelonephritis is an infection of the renal pelvis and interstitium (spaces between the renal tubules). Approximately 85% of pyelonephritis cases are related to *Escherichia coli* (E. coli) bacteria invasions. *Proteus* and *Klebsiella* are less common causative agents; fungal or viral infections are not impossible.

25. A - Rheumatic fever causes lesions to develop on valve leaflets and leads to their inability to function effectively.

26. B - The patient with chronic obstructive pulmonary disease (COPD) has increased difficulty breathing when lying down. His respiratory effort is improved by standing or sitting upright or by having the bed in high Fowler's position.

27. B - IV insulin therapy can cause hypokalemia as insulin moves potassium into the cells with blood sugar. Hypokalemia can lead to cardiac arrhythmias.

28. B - Postoperative DVT (deep vein thrombosis) prophylaxis often involves SCDs while the patient is in bed. The compression device may be discontinued during ambulation, but should then be reapplied when the patient returns to bed.

29. B - Chronic liver failure disrupts the liver's normal use of vitamin K to produce prothrombin (a clotting factor). Consequently, you should monitor the patient for signs of bleeding, including petechiae and ecchymosis.

30. D - Activated partial thromboplastin time (APTT) measures the activity of thromboplastin, which is dependent on intrinsic clotting factors. In hemophilia, the intrinsic clotting factor VIII (antihemophilic factor) is deficient, resulting in a prolonged APTT.

31. B - FSH is a hormone associated with reproduction and the development of sperm in men (spermatogenesis) and eggs (oocytes) in women; it is secreted by the anterior pituitary gland. FSH levels can be used to help determine the reason for a low sperm count in men.

32. A - Dilated, hypertrophic, and restrictive are the three types of cardiomyopathies. There is a cardiac condition called constrictive pericarditis, but this is not a type of cardiomyopathy.

33. B - Pulmonary congestion and edema occur because of fluid extrava-

sation from the pulmonary capillary bed, resulting in difficult breathing (dyspnea). Left-sided heart failure creates a backward effect on the pulmonary system that leads to pulmonary congestion.

34. B - Oxytocin is secreted by the posterior pituitary gland. All three other options are secreted by the anterior pituitary gland.

35. A - Spinal fractures that occur at C7 or above can cause quadriplegia (paralysis of all four limbs). Fractures at T1 or below will cause only paraplegia (paralysis of only the lower two limbs).

36. B - ALS is a neurological disease that destroys motor neurons. ALS will eventually lead to complete paralysis.

37. D - G-tubes are typically large-bore tubes, allowing easy aspiration and delivery of feedings and medications. To avoid mechanical complications, such as the tube becoming obstructed, preventative measures include routinely flushing with 30 mL warm water before and after each medication administration, after checking residuals, after intermittent feedings, and every 4 hours during a continuous feeding.

38. B - The presence of eschar in the lower half of the pressure ulcer makes it impossible to determine if the ulcer is a stage III or a stage IV pressure ulcer, making it necessary to describe it as unstageable.

39. C - During the proliferative phase of the menstrual cycle (days 6 to 14), the endometrium significantly thickens as estrogen levels increase, and cervical mucus becomes more favorable to sperm as it becomes thin, watery, clear, and more alkaline.

40. D - Silent ischemia is ischemia without chest pain. Associated symptoms of the condition are shortness of breath, fatigue, and arrhythmias. It is most commonly found in conjunction with *diabetes mellitus*.

41. C - Cystic fibrosis is a recessive genetic condition. While the nurse may provide some information on the genetic risks, a genetic counselor will be able to better advise the patient on their genetic risks.

42. C - PTU is an anti-thyroid medication that inhibits the synthesis of thyroid hormones; it is used in the treatment of hyperthyroidism.

43. D - Scoliosis refers to a lateral curvature of the spine with vertebral rotation; although the most common curvature is right thoracic, it may occur in any area of the spine (not just thoracic).

44. B - The RYGB is the most commonly performed weight loss surgery. A small stomach pouch is created by dividing the top of the stomach from the rest. The beginning of the small intestine is divided. The distal portion is connected to the newly created pouch, and the proximal end with the attached remainder of the stomach is attached to the small intestine further down to allow for the digestive acids to mix with the food lower in the intestinal tract.

45. C - Erythropoietin, a renal hormone, stimulates bone marrow production of red blood cells (RBCs). This hormone is produced by the kidneys in response to hypoxia and is critical in blood oxygenation. RBCs contain hemoglobin, a protein that is the carrier of oxygen and carbon dioxide.

46. D - BUN is the end product of protein metabolism and is influenced by fluid volume, dietary protein intake, and catabolism. Diabetes mellitus *does not* contribute to an elevated BUN.

47. D - Risk factors for coronary artery disease include; *positive family history of coronary artery disease (CAD)*, *hypertension*, diabetes mellitus, obesity, *male gender*, post-menopausal women, diet high in fat, cholesterol, and sodium, smoking history, sedentary lifestyle, stressful lifestyle, and ethnicity: *African Americans*, Native Americans

48. B - A bronchoscopy involves inserting a scope in the trachea and into the bronchi, allowing direct visualization of these structures. A bronchoscopy typically requires that the patient be intubated.

49. B - This patient who has undergone a thyroidectomy is at risk for developing hypocalcemia (low calcium levels) from inadvertent re-

moval or damage to the parathyroid gland. Chvostek's sign is elicited by tapping the patient's face lightly over the facial nerve, just below the temple.

50.   D - Flexion is the bending of a joint that decreases the angle between two articulating bones. Adduction is the movement of a part toward the midline. Abduction is moving a part of the body away from the midline.

51.   D - Metronidazole (Flagyl) is a commonly used antibiotic to treat or prevent infections (such as *C. diff*), which are related to loss of normal flora in the gut.

52.   C - Pressure ulcers are defined as localized injury to skin and/or underlying tissue usually over a bony prominence, as a result of pressure, or pressure in combination with shear and/or friction. This patient's sacral ulcer should be documented as erythema at this stage since it is superficial and blanchable.

53.   C - Heavy alcohol use has not been shown to be a risk factor for developing bladder cancer.

54.   B - Cardiac tamponade is a medical condition that occurs when fluid fills the pericardial sac, inhibiting the heart's ability to fill and is potentially life-threatening.

55.   D - Bacille Calmette-Guerin vaccine (BCG) is a vaccine against tuberculosis (TB) and people who have been vaccinated with this react to the intradermal test for TB.

56.   A - Hypoglycemia (low blood sugar) is the most frequently seen complication in diabetic patients treated with insulin. It also occurs in patients treated with oral sulfonylureas and combination therapy (insulin and oral medications).

57.   D - Twelve pairs of ribs form the flaring sides of the thorax. Seven pairs of ribs are attached directly to the sternum, while the oth-

er five pairs are false ribs (not directly attached to the sternum). The upper three false ribs connect to the costal cartilages of the ribs just above them. The lower two false ribs usually have no anterior attachment to anchor them in front and so are called floating ribs.

58. B - Ulcerative colitis only affects the large intestine. Ulcerative colitis can lead to bleeding due to mucosal fragility. It is not associated with race, gender, or social class, and it does decrease the absorption of nutrients.

59. A - Hemophilia results from a deficiency of or absent factor VIII (antihemophilic).

60. D - Serum creatinine levels are drawn to help determine the cause and severity of renal failure. Serum creatinine measures the end product of muscle metabolism (protein breakdown in muscle cells).

61. D - The most common symptoms are gastrointestinal and include nausea, vomiting, abdominal pain, and diarrhea.

62. B - The pH is within normal limits (7.35-7.45), but is on the lower end, which, in the context of abnormal PCO2 and HCO3 values, suggests that compensation from acidosis has occurred. The PCO2 is higher than normal limits (35-45 mm Hg), which indicates respiratory acidosis. The HCO3 is slightly higher normal limits (22-26 mEq/L), indicating that it is compensating for the acidosis. This patient has compensated respiratory acidosis.

63. D - Cushing's syndrome is a form of hypercortisolism, resulting from oversecretion of adrenocortical hormones.

64. B - Fat embolism is caused by the release of fat globules into the bloodstream that cause obstructions in blood supply. Fat embolisms occur primarily from fractures of the long bones or of the pelvis. Rib fractures are the least likely of the answer options to cause a fat embolism, as the radius and humerus are both long bones.

65.   B - Indications for enteral feedings include a fairly functional GI tract, inadequate intake for the previous 3 to 5 days (NPO or less than 50% consumed from trays) or already malnourished, and an inability to increase PO nutrients with meals/snacks and oral nutrition supplements (due to the patient not tolerating the increase of PO nutrition).

66.   D - Factor III, also called the "tissue factor," is thromboplastin. It is a proteolytic enzyme, and part of the extrinsic coagulation pathway.

67.   C - Interstitial cystitis is an autoimmune collagen disease which results in inflammation of the bladder wall. It may be non-infectious or abacterial and is most likely to occur in young women (90%-95% of all cases).

68.   A - Warfarin (Coumadin) is an anticoagulant that works by decreasing synthesis of coagulation factors to help prevent blood clots from forming. If taken with steroids, aspirin, glucagons, allopurinol, or metronidazole, warfarin can have an increased action; therefore, it is advised not to take those medications while taking warfarin. Acetaminophen does not interfere with warfarin.

69.   B - The patient with asthma did not achieve relief from shortness of breath after using the bronchodilator and is at risk for respiratory complications. This patient's needs are urgent. The other patients need to be assessed as soon as possible, but none of them is urgent.

70.   D - Antidiuretic hormone (ADH) is synthesized in the hypothalamus, which lies at the base of the brain and regulates endocrine function by the production of regulatory hormones.

71.   D - Patients are evaluated as coping successfully with lifestyle changes after a stroke if they make appropriate lifestyle alterations, accept the assistance of others, and exhibit appropriate social interactions.

72.   D - While the cause of chronic pancreatitis is alcohol abuse in about 80% of cases, this is not always true, and may not be true for this patient.

73. D - First degree (superficial) burns; extend into the epidermis, never blister, are painful, and heal in 3 to 4 days without scarring

74. C - In cancer of the bladder, tumors begin in the transitional cell layer lining the bladder, and this abnormal cell growth and configuration is called dysplasia. This type of cancer may be asymptomatic, but gross, painless hematuria is the first symptom 85% of the time.

75. A - Baroreceptors are located in the carotid bodies and aortic arch; they recognize a decrease in pressure when the body goes into a state of shock.

76. C - Clinical manifestations of chronic bronchitis include:

   - Chronic cough, with production of large amounts of thick, tenacious mucus (not non-productive)
   - Wheezing and rhonchi
   - Cyanosis and hypoxemia that leads to hypercapnia and respiratory acidosis (not respiratory alkalosis)
   - Right-sided congestive heart failure (not left), and pulmonary hypertension

77. D - Primary hyperthyroidism results from hypersecretion of thyroid hormones and is evidenced by increased serum T3 and T4, and decreased serum TSH.

78. D - Possible complications associated with TJA surgery include:

   - Deep vein thrombosis
   - Pulmonary embolism
   - Compartment syndrome
   - Infection
   - Dislocation
   - Joint instability and loosening

Impaired bladder function is not a complication following this type of surgery; it is related to spinal disorders and surgeries.

79. C - Enteral nutrition is *contraindicated* in situations where there is complete intestinal obstruction, prohibiting use of the bowel; parenteral nutrition is indicated in these instances.

80. D - The rule of nines divides body surface area into percentages that, when totaled, equal 100%. According to the rule of nines, the arms account for 9% each, the legs account for 18% each, and the anterior trunk accounts for 18%. Therefore, this client's burns cover 45% of the body surface area.

81. A - As the patient's nurse, you would determine if any allergies to seafood or iodine are present because the dye used for this procedure is iodine-based. The allergic reactions could include hives, itching, rash, tightness in the throat, shortness of breath, and bronchospasm.

82. A - The mean arterial pressure (MAP) is the average arterial pressure during a single cardiac cycle. Diastolic blood pressure (DBP) counts twice as much as systolic blood pressure (SBP) because 2/3 of the cardiac cycle is spent in diastole. A MAP of about 60 is necessary to perfuse the coronary arteries, brain, kidneys.

83. C - COPD is the fourth most common cause of death, and the most common respiratory cause of death in the United States; 16 million individuals in the US have symptomatic COPD. Cigarette smoking is the primary cause of COPD.

84. C - The clavicle, also called the collarbone, is the "brace" that holds the arm away from the thorax.

85. A - Hepatitis A does *not* place the patient at high risk for the future development of hepatic cancer.

86. B - According to the National Pressure Ulcer Advisory Panel (NPUAP), an intact, serum-filled blister is classified as a stage II pressure ulcer.

87. D - The patient with genital herpes should be instructed to avoid sexual intercourse until lesions are completely healed.

88. A - Cardiomyopathy (CMP) is a group of diseases that directly affect the heart muscle, the myocardium. Myopathy may also involve the endocardial and pericardial layers of the heart. It is commonly divided into three categories: Dilated, hypertrophic, and restrictive.

89. A - Hypoxia is the main breathing stimulus for a client with COPD. Supplemental oxygen is used for individuals with severe or progressive hypoxemia. Oxygen use is progressive (during exacerbations only, intermittently, at night, or continuously). Excessive oxygen administration may lead to apnea by removing that stimulus.

90. C - The anterior is the largest lobe of the pituitary gland and secretes several hormones: adrenocorticotropic hormone (ACTH), TSH, luteinizing hormone (LH), follicle-stimulating hormone (FSH), and prolactin.

91. C - Myasthenia gravis is a condition in which nerve signals do not transmit sufficient acetylcholine across the synaptic cleft and the neuromuscular junction or in which there are too few acetylcholine receptors to receive the signals. This results in decreased nerve transmission to muscles, causing weakness. Myasthenia gravis does affect facial muscles, making eating more difficult. This does not, however, typically progress to a condition so severe that eating is not possible.

92. C - The most common presenting symptoms in patients with disorders of the GI tract include; pain, nausea/vomiting, change in bowel pattern, appetite changes, family history, and social history. Evidence of bleeding is an uncommon presenting symptom with gastrointestinal tract disorders and is a cause for concern when present.

93. B - Leukocytes, or white blood cells (WBCs), protect the body from infection. They are subdivided into two forms based on the presence or absence of granules in their cytoplasm: granulocytes and agranulocytes. Neutrophils are granulocytes which serve as the first line of

defense; they act as phagocytes to engulf and absorb invading microorganisms.

94. A - Renin is released in response to hypoperfusion (due to trauma such as hemorrhage, acute heart failure, hypotension from postoperative complications).

95. A - Abdominal aneurysm dissections commonly cause back pain and require emergency treatment. The physician should be notified immediately if severe back pain is experienced by the patient.

96. C - Tumors of the glottis (vocal cords), not the subglottis, are the most common form of laryngeal cancer; subglottic tumors are the least common. Diagnosis of laryngeal cancer is by visualization via laryngoscopy and biopsy (not CT scan).

97. B - DKA is a potentially life-threatening condition that develops when cells in the body are unable to get the sugar (glucose) they need for energy because there is not enough insulin. Signs and symptoms are as follows:

- Hyperglycemia (usually > 250 mg/dl)
- Metabolic acidosis (not alkalosis), characterized by pH less than 7.2
- Dehydration
- Polyuria
- Polydipsia
- Anorexia
- Abdominal pain
- Nausea and vomiting
- Rapid respirations
- Acetone odor to breath
- Weakness
- Warm dry skin
- Tachycardia
- Somnolence
- Coma

98. D - If a patient is actively seizing, intervening could cause harm to yourself or to the patient, as they are not able to control their movements. Ensuring that the patient's environment is safe and that they will not harm themselves during the seizure will be the most useful intervention.

99. B - Ascites, an accumulation of fluid in the abdominal cavity, is a common clinical manifestation in patients with chronic liver failure. Prior to paracentesis, the nurse instructs the patient to void, emptying the bladder, to decrease the chance of puncturing the bladder during the procedure.

100. C - When recognized by T lymphocytes, the foreign invader or material is destroyed. Inflammation and phagocytosis cause destruction of the cell. It takes hours or days for the reaction to reach its peak. Examples of Type IV cell-mediated hypersensitivity reactions include tuberculin skin tests, contact dermatitis, and tissue transplant rejection.

101. C - A patient with a pelvic fracture should not receive an indwelling urinary catheter due to possible urethral trauma that may have occurred during the injury and due to pelvic instability. Kidney function will need to be monitored by other means.

102. B - The apical pulse is located on the chest over the apex of the heart, and best heard with a stethoscope.

103. D - Combat in the armed forces increases the risk of traumatic pneumothorax, not spontaneous pneumothorax.

104. A - Declining pulmonary function is a hallmark of cystic fibrosis. Antibiotics, corticosteroids, and Ivacaftor can slow the progression of lung disease, and mechanical physical therapy devices help CF patients to breathe more easily by loosening and dislodging mucus. For some patients with severe lung damage, lung transplantation is a treatment option.

105. C - Rheumatoid Arthritis is a condition that affects the synovial

membrane and causes stiffness, swelling, severe pain, and deformities that can be serious and disabling; it is a chronic, systemic autoimmune disease with unexplained periods of remission and exacerbation.

106. A - Hyperemesis gravidarum is an obstetric complication and is not associated with PUD. GI hemorrhage, obstruction of the pyloric area, and perforation are all complications of PUD.

107. A - Good sources of vitamin B12 include meats and dairy products.

108. C - Hematuria is often the first symptom of bladder cancer. Pain in the low abdomen and frequent urination are later symptoms. While bladder cancer may initially be asymptomatic, it is likely that some symptoms will develop as the disease progresses.

109. D - Cardiovascular disease kill about 600,000 people in the United States each year.

110. C - A normal PaO2 range is 80-100 mmHg. The patient's ABG indicates that the patient is over oxygenated, which can suppress the respiratory drive in patients with COPD. The patient has mild compensated respiratory acidosis. This is normal for a patient with COPD and does not require any immediate treatment.

111. C - Metformin (Glucophage) is an oral medication used in individuals with type 2 diabetes mellitus; it is classified as a biguanide. It works by increasing insulin sensitivity and decreasing hepatic glucose production by reducing (not increasing) hepatic glycogenolysis and gluconeogenesis.

112. B - Decorticate posturing is an abnormal neurological response in which the arms are bent inward, fists are clenched, and the legs are held out straight.

113. D - The patient has known appendicitis and has symptoms consistent with peritonitis and septic shock. An abdominal CT, while possibly helpful, is not necessary. The patient should receive IV fluids and IV

antibiotics as soon as possible. Earlier surgery may be needed, as the patient's appendicitis is the likely source of the infection and will need to be treated sooner than planned.

114. A - Diabetic ulcers are breakdown of the skin that are commonly caused by diabetic neuropathy and can lead to severe infections and complications that may eventually lead to amputation.

115. C - An elevated serum potassium level may lead to a life-threatening cardiac arrhythmia, which the nurse can detect immediately by palpating the pulse.

116. D - Excitability of the heart is affected by the ionic exchange across cell membranes. Ions which facilitate electrical activity in the heart include sodium, potassium, calcium, and magnesium.

117. D - The five lobar bronchi that diverge from the two mainstream bronchi to enter the lobes of the lungs are partially surrounded by cartilage. The terminal bronchioles do not have cartilage; they depend on elastic recoil of the lungs to maintain airway patency.

118. A - Hormones secreted by a pheochromocytoma can often cause hypertension as a symptom. Pheochromocytomas release epinephrine, norepinephrine, and/or dopamine.

119. B - Dense bones show as white on standard x-ray, providing information about bone deformity, joint congruity, bone density, and calcification, and are the most common diagnostic study used. MRIs, CTs, and bone scans are also diagnostic studies used frequently, but not the most common.

120. A - An ileoanal reservoir is usually created in two stages. First, diseased intestines are removed, and a temporary loop ileostomy is created. Second, the loop ileostomy is closed, and stool goes to the reservoir and out through the anal sphincter, maintaining bowel control and eliminating the need for a permanent ileostomy.

121. D - In liver failure, patients commonly experience metabolic alkalosis. This leads to the electrolyte imbalance hypokalemia (low potassium levels), due to preferential excretion of K+ over H+ to correct the metabolic alkalosis that's occurring within the body.

122. C - Multiple myeloma affects primarily plasma cells in bone marrow.

123. C - Evidence-based guidelines recommend the use of surgical interventions *only when* the patient has bothersome symptoms, complications of benign prostatic hyperplasia, and/or has failed a trial of urinary catheterization.

124. C - Capillaries are the smallest of the body's blood and lymph vessels that make up the microcirculation of the peripheral vascular system. Their thin endothelial linings are only one cell layer thick, with no elastic or muscle tissue present. They help to enable the exchange of water, oxygen, carbon dioxide, and many other nutrients and waste substances between the blood and the tissues surrounding them.

125. D - The FEV1/FVC ratio (forced expiratory volume in 1 second/forced vital capacity) indicates disease progression. As COPD worsens, the ratio of FEV1 to FVC becomes smaller.

126. C - Insulin is required to treat and correct the hyperglycemia causing HHS, not metformin.

127. D - Chronic osteomyelitis is often treated with a combination of surgery and long-term IV antibiotics. A week of oral antibiotics would not be sufficient treatment for chronic osteomyelitis.

128. C - A niacin deficiency does not cause anemia, and giving niacin will not help to treat any kind of anemia.

129. D - PKD is a genetic disease. Asking about family history will enable you to better understand if the patient has genetic risk factors for this condition.

130. C - The definition of mean arterial pressure (MAP) is the average pressure in the arteries. MAP is calculated by using an *weighted* average of the systolic and diastolic blood pressures. The formula is (SBP+2*DBP)/3. A MAP between 100-70 is generally considered healthy, but a MAP that is too high can lead to health problems. Due to the way MAP is calculated, it will never exceed a patient's systolic blood pressure.

131. C - Pulmonary vasculature typically becomes *thicker* (not thinner) and fibrous, which in turn diminishes the effectiveness of gas exchange between alveolus and capillary walls; $pO2$ and $O2$ saturations decline, while pH and $pCO2$ remain the *same* (not increase).

132. A - As insulin moves glucose into the cells, it also moves potassium into the cells, lowering levels of serum potassium.

133. B - Cranial nerve XI is the spinal accessory nerve. It controls movement of the head and shoulder muscles.

134. C - 90% of all upper GI bleeds are associated with peptic ulcers and account for the majority of gastrointestinal hemorrhages. When caring for a patient with a GI bleed, vasomotor instability is the most sensitive indicator of blood loss; changes of 20 bpm or 10 mm Hg systolic indicate a loss of 15%-20% of total blood volume.

135. C - DIC occurs when microclotting increases due to increased thrombin production. This exhausts clotting factors in the blood, making an increased risk for bleeding. While many obstetrical complications can cause DIC, preterm labor is not a potential cause of DIC.

136. C - Chronic pyelonephritis is caused by progressive inflammation leading to fibrosis and scarring; it is also termed chronic interstitial nephritis. The condition is associated with non-bacterial infections and often results from chronic urinary tract obstruction. It may lead to chronic renal failure.

137. D - Patients are NPO (nothing by mouth) for 6-12 hours before the

procedure to reduce the risk of aspiration. Following cardiac catheterization, the patient is kept in bed with no bending of the extremity used for the procedure for *24 hours*.

138. D - Transudative pleural effusion occurs when fluid accumulates in the pleural space as a result of increased hydrostatic pressure or low plasma proteins. Congestive heart failure (CHF) is the most common cause of transudative pleural effusions. Less common causes include chronic kidney disease, liver failure, and malignancy.

139. B - The hemoglobin A1C measures glucose accumulation on red blood cells, which have a lifespan of about three months. At the end of their lifespan, red blood cells are removed from circulation by the spleen. A patient who has a history of splenectomy will have an elevated A1C due to the increased lifespan of the red blood cells, and the data obtained will not be usable.

140. A - Seizures may occur at a slightly higher incidence in people with multiple sclerosis (MS), but are not nearly as commonly associated with MS as the other three symptoms.

141. A - A patient with acute pancreatitis is to be started on parenteral nutrition (feeding by intravenous route, bypassing the usual process of eating and digestion). Contraindications for parenteral nutrition include a functional gastrointestinal tract, no venous access, and health care directives that decline parenteral nutrition.

142. D - According to the National Pressure Ulcer Advisory Panel, Stage III pressure ulcers present with full thickness tissue loss involving subcutaneous tissue; bone, tendon, or muscle is not exposed. Slough (yellow, tan, gray, green, or brown in color) may be present but does not obscure the depth of tissue loss.

143. D - Specific gravity can be measured by dipstick, refractometer, or urinometer, with the dipstick being the most common and urinometer being the least common.

144. B - Angiography allows for direct visualization and evaluation of the blood flow through the coronary arteries, making it the most accurate and comprehensive method for diagnosing myocardial infarction.

145. D - The patient's slow rate of breathing will cause the patient to retain carbon dioxide and will also lead to hypoxia. The ABG will likely show an elevated carbon dioxide level. This will cause the pH to drop. The bicarbonate levels are controlled by the kidneys and respond more slowly. If the patient was in this condition for several weeks, which would be very unlikely, the kidneys would increase the levels of bicarbonate to compensate for the acidosis caused by the carbon dioxide, bringing the pH into a normal range. Because this is an acute condition, the patient would be uncompensated, and the patient would be developing acidosis that is related to a respiratory cause.

146. C - Tolbutamide (Orinase) generally works in the body for 6 to 12 hours.

147. C - Corticosteroid therapy for OA includes intra-articular injections (administered directly into a joint) for best effect; these injections are often used to treat inflamed joints.

148. B - A volvulus is twisting of the intestines and may require surgery. A patient with a volvulus should not have anything to eat or drink until the volvulus is resolved, both because food will not be able to pass through the intestines and because surgery is possible.

149. B - Because these three pressure ulcers are separated by intact skin, they should be documented as three distinct pressure ulcers, even though they are in the same area. The tunneling that exists should be noted in the assessment of each of the two pressure ulcers that it affects. It would not be likely that a determination could be made about the origin of the tunneling if it connects two pressure ulcers.

150. D - The cortex of the kidney is the outermost layer; it is located just under the tightly adhering fibrous capsule.

CPSIA information can be obtained
at www.ICGtesting.com
Printed in the USA
LVHW062321310821
696551LV00002B/88